SCIENTIFIC AIDS IN HOSPITAL DIAGNOSIS

[Conference on]

SCIENTIFIC AIDS IN HOSPITAL DIAGNOSIS

Edited by
J. P. Nicholson
*Westminster Hospital
London, England*

RC71
A1
C668
1976

PLENUM PRESS · NEW YORK AND LONDON

Library of Congress Cataloging in Publication Data

Conference on Scientific Aids in Hospital Diagnosis, Oxford, 1975.
    Scientific aids in hospital diagnosis.

    "Proceedings of a Conference on Scientific Aids in Hospital Diagnosis organized by the United Kingdom Liaison Committee for Sciences Allied to Medicine and Biology at Oxford, England, April, 1975."
    Includes index.
    1. Diagnosis—Congresses. 2. Hospitals—Diagnostic services—Congresses. I. Nicholson, John Philip. II. UK Liaison Committee for Sciences Applied to Medicine and Biology. III. Title [DNLM: 1. Diagnosis—Congresses. 2. Diagnosis, Computer assisted—Congresses. 3. Diagnosis, Laboratory—Congresses. 3. Radiography—Congresses. WB141 C747s 1975]
RC71.C668 1975   616.07'5'028   76-15409
ISBN 0-306-30938-6

Proceedings of a Conference on Scientific Aids in Hospital Diagnosis
organized by the United Kingdom Liaison Committee for Sciences Allied
to Medicine and Biology at Oxford, England, April, 1975

© 1976 Plenum Press, New York
A Division of Plenum Publishing Corporation
227 West 17th Street, New York, N.Y. 10011

All rights reserved

No part of this book may be reproduced, stored in a retrieval system, or transmitted, in any form or by any means, electronic, mechanical, photocopying, microfilming, recording, or otherwise, without written permission from the Publisher

Printed in the United States of America

Preface

This volume contains the Proceedings of a Conference on Scientific Aids in Hospital Diagnosis held at Oxford in April 1975. The Conference, organised on inter-disciplinary lines, was the fourth to be organised by the U. K. Liaison Committee for Sciences allied to Medicine and Biology (SAMB).

The subject matter is divided into six sections: Investigations in Pathology, Radiation Diagnostics, New Diagnostic Techniques in Special Departments, Clinical Measurements in Wards, Coordination and Communication of Results, and finally Ergonomic Contributions to Medical Diagnosis. Session IV may be found of particular interest as it puts the point of view of the nurses who have to operate so many of the new machines and pieces of equipment, often under stressful conditions.

We were fortunate in having as our Guest Speaker, Sir George Godber, Former Chief Medical Officer to the Department of Health and Social Security. Sir George's career has spanned the time during which very many scientific technqiues have been introduced into medicine and few people could be better qualified to give an overall picture of the present situation.

J. P. NICHOLSON
(Honorary Secretary, SAMB)

Contents

Preface . . . .

PART I

INVESTIGATIONS IN PATHOLOGY

(Chairman: Mr. T. S. Lansley,
East Ham Memorial Hospital)

Automation in Pathology 3
   Robert George Fewell

Screening for Disease 9
   Peter Wilding

Centralisation of Pathology Laboratories 19
   R. J. Mills and J. Dawson

Keeping a Balance - Specialised Analyses 29
   W. H. P. Lewis

Laboratory Diagnosis of Genetic Problems 35
   L. J. Butler

PART II

RADIATION DIAGNOSTICS

(Chairman: Mr. R. C. T. Buchan,
Medical Physics Department, General Hospital, Plymouth)

Provision of a Mammography Service 57
   M. Davison

Ultrasonic Diagnostics: Capabilities of Present
        Systems   63
    P. N. T. Wells

Radionuclide Imaging - A Quick Scan Through   73
    J. A. McIntosh

Thermography in the Investigation of Breast Cancer   79
    A. L. Evans, W. B. James, and M. Davison

Perspectives in Radiodiagnosis   85
    Louis Kreel

PART III

NEW DIAGNOSTIC TECHNIQUES IN SPECIAL DEPARTMENTS

(Chairman: Sir Roger Bannister,
National Hospital, Queen Square, London)

Monitoring the EEG in Liver Disease   95
    B. MacGillivray, D. Wadbrook, and P. M. Quilter

The Use of EEG Telemetry and Videorecording in
        the Differential Diagnosis of Fits 107
    A. N. Bowden

Haemodynamic Assessment by Transcutaneous
        Aortovelography in Intensive Therapy 109
    J. Beardshaw and G. Hanson

Design Principles of the E. M. I. Scanner 119
    G. N. Hounsfield

Practical Experience with the E. M. I. Scanner 131
    J. Gawler

Visually Evoked Cortical Potentials in
        Neurological Diagnosis 139
    A. M. Halliday

Peripherally Evoked Spinal Cord Potentials in
        Neurological Diagnosis 155
    D. G. Small

CONTENTS

PART IV

CLINICAL MEASUREMENTS IN WARDS

(Chairman: Miss Geraldine Willman,
Coronary Care Unit, Royal Infirmary, Manchester)

Guest Lecture 167
   Sir George Godber

Nurse - Patient - Computer Interaction 175
   Gillian Tobin

The Patient and the Machine 179
   C. M. Roberts

Keeping the Balance Between Basic and Technical
           Nursing 185
   Aideen Phillips

PART V

COORDINATION AND COMMUNICATION OF RESULTS

(Chairman: Dr. B. Barber,
Operational Research Unit, London Hospital)

Chairman's Introduction 193
   Barry Barber

Review of Medical Linguistics in Computing
        with Special Reference to "Mumps" 197
   D. E. Clark, T. C. Sharpe, and A. J. Duxbury

Progress Towards Health Information Systems 207
   Michael Alderson

Progress Towards Computer-Aided Medical
          Decision-Making 211
   F. T. de Dombal

The London Hospital Computer System - A Case Study 215
   W. Abbott

Towards Microfilm Systems in the Health Service 223
   E. J. Steadman

Multi-Image Storage 231
   J. Hambleton

PART VI

ERGONOMIC CONTRIBUTIONS TO MEDICAL DIAGNOSIS

(Chairman: Mr. C. J. A. Andrews,
Department of Biological Sciences, Napier College of
Commerce and Technology, Edinburgh)

Chairman's Introductory Statement 241
    Clive J. A. Andrews

Industrial Experience of Ergonomics as Applied
        to Clinical Diagnosis 243
    G. J. Gillies

The Rationale of Clinical Problem Solving 251
    Donald L. Crombie

The Ergonomics of Clinical Diagnosis in an
        Intensive Care Ward 267
    D. E. M. Taylor

Index 281

PART I

Investigations in Pathology

AUTOMATION IN PATHOLOGY

Robert George Fewell

The London Hospital, London

The problem of handling an ever increasing number of analyses in pathology is common to all laboratories and disciplines. The nature of the problem varies within the discipline and has necessarily meant differing developmental approaches. For instance in clinical chemistry a much earlier start was made than in some other fields toward mechanised procedures to improve speed of analysis with accuracy and precision, particularly in fields where chemical stability is evident; e.g. it is possible to estimate substances like potassium very easily but some of the more fickle enzyme systems are more difficult; standard condition of assay for the former are easily met but for the latter are much more demanding. Clinical chemistry today remains in the forefront of automated processes illustrating the point that any repetitive process can and will be mechanised given money and time for development. Whilst the chemists have their problems they are seemingly insignificant when compared with say the medical microbiologist. In this area some mechanisation is possible e.g. in media kitchens for dispensing culture media; some attempts have been made to mechanise seeding of culture media with specimen material with limited success. Identification of microbes still remains a highly sophisticated problem which can only yet be tackled by the most highly developed mechanism known - the human brain. Attempts are being made to tackle the problem and some of the newer techniques available such as gas chromatography are making a valuable contribution. However full automation seems a long way off.

In histopathology many of the repetitive processes needed for the preparation of material for microscopical analysis have been mechanised for a goodly number of years. The fixation of tissue and some staining processes are easily adapted to automatic tissue processors and staining machines. The interpretive study of the end product, the stained section, still remains for the human eye and brain and there seems little hope in the near future of machinery taking over this function.

However, in all disciplines there is one area where full automation can be achieved, depending upon how much money is available, - that of data processing. Before going further with this area I would wish to put before you evidence of how one other pathology discipline, so far unmentioned, has developed, and is still developing, methods for repetitive and often boring procedures which enable accuracy, precision and speed to be achieved which the human element cannot match. With the help of some slides perhaps this development is best illustrated.

Firstly the problems must be posed and the answer sought. A stained film of human blood will show three elements, the erythrocytes, leucocytes and platelets. Numerical haematology demands accurate counting of these elements which may be increased or decreased in numbers in disease processes. Additionally the haemoglobin content of the erythrocytes needs to be measured. All these parameters were crudely measured until sophisticated electronic apparatus became available. The haemoglobin was measured two decades or so ago by matching with a coloured glass standard and the cellular elements laboriously counted by eye under a microscope having been set up on an accurately ruled glass slide, the counting chamber. Modern day practice determines colour photoelectrically and the counting process is now done electronically. Both of these developments revolutionised haematological measurement and such is the speed and refinement of the mechanised equipment in use today the older manual methods cannot be remotely compared.

There remains one problem; the differential leucocyte count. Developments are taking place in this field and two current lines of investigation into the problem hold promise. One system attempts automatic screening with visual display and computer printout and another attempts to identify cells by differential staining also with printout. It may be fairly said that at present recognising normal cells is theoretically a workable proposition but recognising the abnormal is much more difficult. Classification of abnormal cells is still a matter for the human eye and brain.

In many hospital laboratories blood group serology and transfusion departments are part of the haematology service although in the larger units they tend to be separate entities. Even where this is so staff both medical and technical need to gain experience in both fields for examination purposes, particularly at primary qualification level.

In the modern blood transfusion and serology department ABO and Rhesus typing of red blood cells may now be carried out by machine with considerable speed and a great degree of accuracy. Basically the admixture of reagents is undertaken in a continous line system and the resultant reaction or non-reaction aliquoted on to high grade absorbent paper. The results are recorded according to the appearance of "granularity" or "clumping" of the cells as opposed to a "smooth" appearance.

I hope these slides have illustrated how in haematology and blood group serology increasing workloads are being handled. However in spite of the sophistication of some of these machines it should be remembered they are only as good as the operating programme prepared for them. Clearly patient identification is all important.

It is obvious if they are not calibrated correctly the whole exercise is useless. Rigid quality control and proficiency monitoring are essential. And in case of breakdown a back-up system must be available.

DATA PROCESSING

Inevitably when the machine has done its job the results produced must then be returned to the patients' notes. Automated equipment produces either digital or analogue information and in either case further processing may be necessary before the results are incorporated in the case notes. Various methods are available depending upon the situation but suffice it to say that most departments have a local, that is in-the-laboratory, process and the printed end result is issued from there, suitably validated. However real time on line systems are being attempted.

A completely automated system should have three main features:

1) a requesting service for medical staff.

2) a data processing system on line real time.

3) a reporting system.

The first request is obtained by means of visual display units (VDU) situated at points throughout the hospital, wards, clinics, etc. By using a set procedure medical staff can effect requests for laboratory investigation for anything they require. As far as possible the requests are programmed and by a digital system discipline specific requests are activated. The request is then printed by a line printer either in the laboratory office or other suitable point.

Once specimen and form is received in the laboratory the examination can be carried out. The results are held in an intermediate store to await validation. Much of the information will have been picked up direct from the automated apparatus, the results being known to the laboratory by teletype alongside the apparatus. Quality control and proficiency monitoring can be controlled by the operator through the computer to previously defined limits.

The generated information once validated can be issued as hard copy from a central point and distributed thence to the patients' notes. These reports can be accumulative and this particular facility enables the clinical staff at a glance to see the progress of the patient in those areas where sequential requests have been made.

In addition to the hard copy all results for a patient are available on a VDU during his stay in hospital, and for a week after discharge. They are then archived on tape and may be recalled at a later date if required.

HOW FAR DO WE GO?

I have outlined an involved system, which given dedication and finance has many advantages. At best a result of an investigation can be before the clinical staff in minutes either validated or not. At worst when the computer is down delays can be enormous due to requests in the pipe-line which may be held up or indeed lost altogether due to the inability to print. One could go on elaborating pros and cons for the system I have outlined; all systems of data-processing can be so appraised. How far do we go? In my view as far as possible toward the ideal situation of full computerisation although I realise that the diverse demands of pathology make it an expensive exercise. However given the dedication of all staff (a slow process) the advantages outweigh the disadvantages. Perfection is not for this world although this is no reason why we should not strive to get as near as possible along the road toward it. Nirvana is a long way off and the fears of some that individuality is being destroyed and absorption into one whole attempted are in my view groundless. We must always push forward and, in the field of pathology, progress is paramount - for the happiness and health of us all.

SCREENING FOR DISEASE

PETER WILDING

DEPARTMENT OF CLINICAL CHEMISTRY

QUEEN ELIZABETH MEDICAL CENTRE, BIRMINGHAM

It is extremely difficult to present an interesting lecture on the principles of biochemical profiling for workers currently engaged in screening or in clinical laboratory work. Obviously, many of you realise the reasons and justification for these procedures and hence it will be my aim in the next 20 minutes to merely outline the principles of profiling as I see them and to illustrate these principles with examples of my own experience.

Obviously the motive for profiling is dependent on the population being investigated. In the well population the primary aim is the detection of pre-symptomatic disease. In practice, this results in a small yield and published figures would indicate a yield of unsuspected abnormality in 5 - 15% of the patients being investigated.

For the hospital population the motive is that of improving diagnosis or in the control or monitoring of treatment. Many hospitals who introduced biochemical profiling as a method of screening patients at admission, now realise that it is also a convenient method of follow-up for patients and of simplifying the pattern of work in the laboratory.

There is little doubt that certain tests are worthy of inclusion in biochemical profiles. These tests are usually associated with treatable conditions. Examples are serum calcium - for the detection of unsuspected hyperparathyroidism and cholesterol and triglyceride assays - for the detection and monitoring of hyperlipoproteinaemia. Most clinical chemists would also argue that certain liver function tests should be included. However,

TABLE 1

BIOCHEMICAL PROFILES - CURRENT TESTS

Glucose	Iron
Uric Acid	Potassium
Alkaline Phosphatase	Total Lipids
Alanine Transaminase	Gamma Glutamyl Transpeptidase
Globulin	Creatinine
Sodium	Calcium
Triglycerides	Aspartate Transaminase
Chloride	Albumin
Urea	Iron Binding Capacity
Phosphorus	Cholesterol
Bilirubin	Bicarbonate
Lactate Dehydrogenase	5' Nucleotidase
P.B.I.	Thyroxine

there are also those tests which require to be included because they confirm or eliminate the diagnosis of common disease, even though the disease may be treatable.

The economic justification of profiling can be argued from many angles. Time-saving derives from reduction in the period of hospitalisation and reduction in the use of man power in the laboratory. Capital costs associated with profiling are, in many instances, considerable and many argue that the purchase of large expensive items of automation is a strong reason for not embarking on profiling of any population. On the other hand, items of equipment, albeit expensive, may in the long term be cheaper than many individual items of analysing equipment. Operating costs involved in profiling may be considerable. The operating costs are function of formulation of the profiles used and the simple exclusion of one determination may cause great reductions in the cost of reagents. For example the exclusion of uric acid and alanine transferase assays from the most commonly used battery of tests are likely to reduce the cost of reagents to a quarter.

Table 1 includes those tests which are generally considered for inclusion in biochemical profiles both in screening centres and in hospitals. Clinical chemists will argue for long periods as to which of these tests are essential components of an efficient screening project. The economic restrictions and technical complexity of a system which included all these tests would be considerable.

A more realistic group of tests (Table 2) probably fulfils the requirements for most screening centres dealing with ambulant patients. Many may argue that I have omitted tests which they

TABLE 2

ESSENTIAL TESTS FOR WELL POPULATION SCREENING

1. Glucose
2. Urea or creatinine
3. Uric acid
4. Calcium
5. Alkaline phosphatase
6. Aspartate transaminase
7. Total protein
8. Cholesterol
9. Triglycerides

consider essential to any screening programme. Nevertheless, it is my experience that tests not included in this list do little to add to the efficiency of a programme aimed to detect pre-symptomatic diseases. However, a laboratory performing biochemical profiling with this group of tests would be required to perform numerous additional assays in the event that abnormality was found or suspected. High on the list of priorities for the second line of tests are the enzymes 5' nucleotidase and gamma glutamyl transpeptidase and facilities for electrophoresis for proteins and lipoproteins. Practically, there is little justification (clinically or economically) for using 12 or 20 tests just because analytical channels are available on a large analyser. The influence of instrument manufacturers on the formulation of test profiles is too great and the selection of tests should always be made after due consideration of the population under study. Ideally the formulation of the profile should be adjusted for each case under investigation. This type of facility is a feature of the many new analysers or those currently under development.

Certain tests which are employed routinely in the hospital clinical laboratory have little place in screening the well population. The obvious tests, in my opinion, which may be identified in this way are serum albumin, sodium and potassium. Albumin plays an important role in the hospital clinical laboratory, but is rarely abnormal in the ambulant patients. This is also true of the electrolytes sodium and potassium. For economic reasons, as well as the practical reason of not creating additional unnecessary of confusing data, care should be taken to prevent unnecessary duplication. For example the assay of urea AND creatinine or aspartate transferase AND alanine transferase should only be embarked on when clinically and economically justified.

In our laboratory we have carried out several studies in an attempt to eliminate those tests which merely duplicate information.

FIGURE 1

BIOCHEMICAL PROFILES - DECEMBER 1972

    Total number   1714
    Actual patients   1035
    Ala-T (SGPT) assays   868
    LDH assays   996

FIGURE 2

ABNORMAL ALA-T (SGPT) VALUES

Number of patients with values mean + 2 S.D. = 92

Number of patients with:
  Alk. Phos. $\not> 24$ (3-14))
  Asp-T (SGOT) $\not> 60$ (30)) = 24

$\therefore$ 868 assays $\longrightarrow$ <u>24</u>

ABNORMAL LDH VALUES

Number of patients with values mean + 2 S.D. = 79

Number of patients with:
  Alk. Phos. $\not> 24$ (3-14))
  Asp-T (SGOT) $\not> 60$ (30)) = 34

$\therefore$ 996 assays $\longrightarrow$ <u>34</u>

As a result of these studies we have eliminated the assays of alanine transferase and lactate dehydrogenase from our biochemical profile.

    Figures 1 and 2 show that major abnormality was only detected in the assays for alanine transferase and lactate dehydrogenase in 92 and 79 patients respectively. However, in only 24 patients were the alanine transferase results not associated with significant increases in the alkaline phosphatase or aspartate transferase results and similarly in only 34 patients were the lactate dehydrogenase values not associated with similar abnormalities of alkaline phosphatase and aspartate transferase.

    Figure 3 shows that for most of the patients in whom the abnormalities were detected, the finding was of little clinical value.

FIGURE 3

UNEXPLAINED RESULTS

	Total Unexplained	Notes Located	Remainder Unexplained
Ala-T (SGPT)	24	16	9
LDH	34	24	10

    Chemotherapy
    ESR > 60 mm/hr
    Terminal carcinoma
    Renal transplants
    Died within a few days
    > 80 years

The new developments in biochemical profiling are perhaps of greater interest to this audience. These might be divided in the following way:

    New tests
    Computer diagnosis
    Discriminate/cluster analysis

New tests which have been introduced recently and which probably justify inclusion in a screening profile would certainly include assay for gamma glutamyl transpeptidase. Its role in the detection of alcoholism makes the test valuable in most countries even though there are other conditions or drugs which cause elevation of the enzyme. In the past, assays for thyroid function have been restricted to protein bound iodine. Newer, simpler and more specific methods for thyroid hormones now make inclusion of such tests highly desirable.

The collection of large amounts of data on single patients may easily be regarded as insignificant if no major abnormality is detected for any one parameter. This attitude derives from our inability to comprehend more than three dimensions. It is possible that a biochemical profile may still indicate disease, possibly pre-symptomatic, even though no major abnormality is present.

We have attempted to enter this field of investigation by examining both the role of the computer in diagnosis and also by studying the value of discriminant or cluster analyses of results obtained by biochemical profiling. Our first attempt was to test the simple approach of Hobbie and Reece (1). These authors have suggested a method of analyses which results in a list of diagnostic possibilities. The computer considers abnormal values only and then compares these abnormalities with a library of associated

TABLE 3

COMPARISON OF RESULTS OF CORRECT AND INCORRECT DIAGNOSES BY
A COMPUTER AND FOUR CLINICIANS

	Right Answers		Wrong Answers		No Diagnosis Possible	
	No.	%	No.	%	No.	%
Computer	36.5	42.5	45.5	53.0	4.0	4.5
Dr. A	26.0	30.0	12.0	14.0	48.0	56.0
Dr. B	21.5	25.0	14.5	17.0	50.0	58.0
Dr. C	30.0	35.0	22.0	25.5	34.0	39.5
Dr. D	30.5	35.5	16.5	19.0	39.0	45.5

conditions. Our experience is summarised in Tables 3 and 4. We tested the Hobbie and Reece program using results from 200 patients whose diagnosis was clearly defined.

The results indicate that major deficiencies are still present in the Hobbie and Reece program and its approach to computer diagnosis. More recently we have attempted to investigate the role of discriminant or cluster analyses in patients with rheumatoid arthritis. We posed the following questions:-

1. Are biochemical profiles of patients with rheumatoid arthritis different?
2. Are there biochemical or haematological parameters which are better in disease for diagnostic purposes than those in current use?
3. Are the biochemical profiles of rheumatoid arthritis patients receiving various drugs different?

TABLE 4

COMPUTER DIAGNOSIS OF MYOCARDIAL INFARCTION IN 20 PATIENTS

RESULT	NO. OF PATIENTS
Computer and clinicians* correct	9
Computer only correct	2
Clinicians* only correct	3
Computer and clinicians* both wrong	6

* The results obtained by the clinicians were considered collectively.

SCREENING FOR DISEASE

Our work to date suggests that there are detectable differences in the profiles of patients with this disease and the major differences are detected in albumin and bilirubin. Our work further indicates that activity of the disease is better assessed by diminution in the albumin value than it is by the ESR measurement. The differences in the patients receiving different drugs are illustrated in Figure 4, which demonstrates that using the discriminant or cluster type analyses, patients receiving aspirin, steroids or a mixture of both can be differentiated. This work is continuing.

The evaluation of biochemical profiling is an important exercise for all those engaged in using this technique. However,

FIGURE 4

DIFFERENTIATION OF PATIENTS WITH RHEUMATOID ARTHRITIS RECEIVING VARIOUS DRUGS

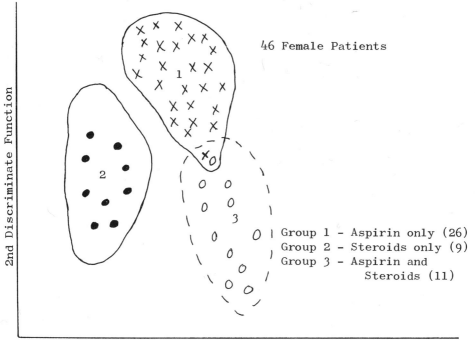

NOTE: Isolation of Group 1 effected mainly by W.B.C. (↓)
Isolation of Group 2 effected mainly by cholesterol (↑) and calcium (↓)

in order to evaluate profiling it is imperative that good data be available, but data is only good when it is accessible. Furthermore, when attempting to evaluate the data it is important that only simple questions are posed as all too frequnetly the answer to complex questions is too complex to understand. Finally, it is imperative that long-term assessment of biochemical profiling also be carried out. Table 5 summarises the work in our department by my colleagues who have attempted to follow-up, over a period of 5 years, unexpected, unexplained abnormalities which were detected when biochemical profiles were performed on patients admitted to medical and surgical wards of our hospital.

TABLE 5

FIVE YEAR FOLLOW-UP OF PROFILE

CATEGORY	DESCRIPTION	NO. OF PATIENTS
1	Unidentified symptomatic	1 (0.5%)
2	Pre-symptomatic	3 (1.5%)
3	Patients with results eventually explained	74 (37%)
4	Results which were normal on repeat	71 (35%)
5	Persistent unexplained abnormal results	7 (3.5%)
6	Unclassified: Persistent high cholesterol	7 (3.5%)
	Lower serum iron	11 (5.5%)
7	Died	7 (3.5%)
	Unable to attend	19 (9.5%)
	TOTAL	200

(Bradwell, A.R., Carmalt, M.H.B., Whitehead, T.P.)
(THE LANCET, November 2, 1974, p.1071)

REFERENCE

1. REECE, R.L., HOBBIE, R.K.: Computer evaluation of chemistry values A reporting and diagnostic aid. Am. J. Clin. Pathol. 57: 664-675, 1972.

Discussion

Dr Barber (London): I think that we should not be worrying about computers but rather about the mathematics. It is not a question of what the clinician said versus what the computer said but what are the underlying assumptions in either case and which are correct. The fundamental matters are those of mathematical modelling not how the sums were done. Some years ago while visiting Dr Albert Casey in Birmingham, Alabama I was able to see the biochemical profiles he had created in his laboratory based from a large, basically outpatient, population. This work was of much greater general interest than the material from most hospital laboratories because the ill population is seen in its context of a substantially well population. Computer facilities in conjunction with automated apparatus now enable us to screen populations effectively. This must not be done thoughtlessly, but the re-organised Health Service starts with the concept of care for a defined population and it seems to me logical that one should seek to ascertain some information about the population in health as in sickness. Certainly, one may expect that decision criteria worked out for sick populations in hospital will be inappropriate for action on well populations outside hospital but that is no argument against collecting the evidence now that it is technically feasible. The move in the re-organised service towards a consideration of the health of the population rather than the management of institutions is a welcome one and definitely overdue.

Dr Wilding: The problem of screening is that it gives rise to a bottomless pit of expense and patients tend to use it as a weapon. One just cannot contemplate screening of the world population. It can be justified once the patient goes to their general practitioner but the existing laboratories in this country could not possibly perform all the necessary tests if a general screening approach were contemplated. Screening must be directed from within the hospital but must come outside the hospital to obtain relevant information.

Dr Barber: This is only true if widespread information were accepted as an immediate cost on National Health Service funding.

There is no reason why it should not be justified as a controlled clinical trial with a pilot population to assess the effects on the health of the population experimentally. Indeed, this is just the sort of pioneering development that should be centrally funded to improve population health instead of simply giving up because it might be too expensive, or too time and resource consuming.

Dr Tárnoky (Reading): I think that when a patient goes to a general practitioner he goes with a definite complaint. The general practitioner will then decide what tests to request for his differential diagnosis, and these tests are likely to form part of a group of tests: a sub-profile, routinely carried out by the local laboratory. To do this type of profile or sub-profile seems to me to be justified; it would be cheaper to do it at the GP stage than to admit the patient to hospital.

Dr Lewis (London): There are two points that I should like to make: (i) How do we decide which results are abnormal? The normal ranges are usually established on a population of less than 50 and the number of patients' results compared against this normal range runs into many thousands. Normal variation will ensure that a proportion of results will be outside the normal range defined in this way, and these individuals are probably not abnormal in any way. And (ii) individuals will occur who give results which will be the normal pattern for them and which results from the enormous amount of variability that occurs in human populations.

Dr Mills (Southend): The laboratory cannot work in isolation and disregard the clinician. It must provide clinicians with meaningful results within as short a time as possible, and such results must be iterpreted against a background of normality for that laboratory.

Dr Healey (Barnsley): I was fascinated by the table Dr Wilding showed comparing the accuracy of the pathologist's diagnosis compared with a computer programme. Many similar trials in diagnostic radiology, my own specialty, in eleven countries throughout Europe, in the United States, and at some centres in the British Isles, have shown a remarkable consistency in the "error rate" of usually about 25%. This has been quoted against my specialty on several occasions by my own colleagues and I shall be delighted in future to quote Dr Wilding's figures showing up to 75% "error rate" for pathologists. I arrived at this last figure by adding together the "wrong diagnosis" and the "don't know" categories. This last category fascinated me, since radiologists, in general, cannot report "don't know". When assessing "error rates" it is assumed that all the information is available on the film or series of films being considered and the "error rate" is assessed according as one over-diagnoses or under-diagnoses.

CENTRALISATION OF PATHOLOGY LABORATORIES

R.J. Mills   and   the late J. Dawson

Principal Biochemist   Consultant Chemical Pathologist

Southend General Hospital   St. Andrews Hospital

Centralisation is a highly emotive word. In most peoples' mind it represents a force which they cannot control, and which is going to alter their working lives. Individuals believe it will be imposed for economic reasons, thus leading to fears of job security and loss of senior positions. Equally, the arguments raised against centralisation, are altruistic, often that the service to patients and clinicians will be diminished. Whether the present level of service is based on correct assumptions is not considered. An investigatory service must be firmly based on real need and must not occur because Pathology has just grown like Topsy. We have never questioned by experiment, the sort of service we are at present providing or indeed should provide.

We consider centralisation initially is about the creation of scientifically viable units which can make real contributions to patient welfare. Obviously this should be done as economically as possible.

Secondly if a centralisation scheme was found unacceptable to technical staff and clinicians after experiment and discussion of the possible benefits, such as increased versatility of investigatory procedures, and decreased turn-round time of results, then such a scheme deserves to fail and would not be implemented. Any scheme however does require experimentation with a dispassionate appraisal of the results before either adoption or rejection. Lay administrators can assess the economic aspects and if the price is too high the scheme will and should fail anyway.

Thirdly, any experiments about providing a service must not be hampered by euclidian lines drawn on maps as administrative boundaries. Such lines can, under some circumstances, take on all the power of electrified barbed wire fences. Administrative processes should run a laboratory service devised by the individuals providing the Pathology service, and we should not have to run a service created by an administration. Thus to us the concept of administrative convenience is not viable.

Fourthly, we no longer consider the concept of pathology as a single discipline to be useful. The separate disciplines of pathology should be allowed to organise themselves separately. Thus the widely different technologies and methods of work organisation each one has, can be considered, whilst providing for the development of individual disciplines. We may now debate whether Pathology Departments as such, should be constructed in toto, or whether the siting and building of each discipline should be considered separately.

Finally, all of the discussion on laboratory centralisation now assumes a dichotomy, between a consultative function of individuals associated with laboratories, and the function of the laboratory as a data-producing organisation. Indeed, in some disciplines, centralisation may accelerate acceptance of the concept that medically trained personnel, at present in laboratories, should have a much greater clinical role. Thus they should be based in hospitals, and have only a minor laboratory role. On the other hand the laboratory should be organised and administered by non-medical personnel. This, of course, raises the problem of who should control laboratories engaged in haematology, microbiology and clinical chemistry.

We will now investigate a situation in which various levels of centralisation have occurred, examine some of the factors which caused these to occur, and consider some of the benefits that have accrued.

Figure 1 illustrates a schematic diagram of the Hospitals in a given geographic space, roughly bounded by the HM.70/50 definition of a centralisable area as having a 20 miles radius or being within 1 hours travelling time by van. This area includes a lot of Hospitals and if geriatric and community Hospitals had been included there would be even more. Of course none of the latter have laboratory facilities, nor have they ever had them. The diagram encompasses five separate health districts in two separate Area Health Authorities. The separate Health Districts comprise, Hospitals S and R; A, B, O, and SO; BO, C and J; which three districts constitute part of one Area Health Authority and the two districts constituting a totally separate Area Health

CENTRALIZATION OF PATHOLOGY LABORATORIES

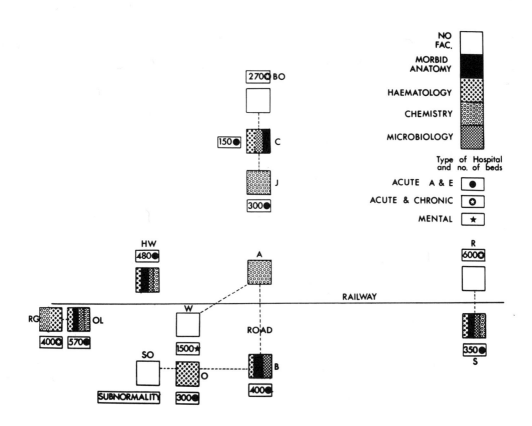

FIGURE I

Schematic Map of hospitals within a given geographic area (approximately 15 mile radius centred on A). Hospitals R and S in one Health District area approximately 3 miles apart, hospitals BO, C and J are in another Health District BO to C is 4 miles and J to A a further $1\frac{1}{2}$ miles. In a third Health District, A is 6 miles from B whilst O is a further 8 miles and SO an additional $5\frac{1}{2}$ miles away. Hospital W, 7 miles away from A, which has always done the work for W, is in a separate Area Health Authority. These three districts constitute part of one Health Authority, J is $6\frac{1}{2}$ miles away from A by road. Hospitals RG and OL are 1 mile apart in one Health District and HW in the other Health District of a separate Area Health Authority.

Authority encompass Hospitals HW and W in one district and RG and OC in the other.

We will now consider the organisation in the district comprising of Hospital's A, B, O and SO: Chemistry is entirely sited at Hospital A and has no "hot labs" in the other two. Histology is at B with facilities for P.M.'s at only Hospital O. Bacteriology is also sited at Hospital B but has no facilities in the other two Hospitals, whilst Haematology is in Hospital O with a transfusion hot lab at B. This District also draws in work from a large Mental Hospital W, and a large subnormality Hospital SO. So here we have individual disciplines of pathology each operating separately and having more laboratory space than they would have if all were represented in every Hospital. As the work and total technical staff for a discipline are concentrated we are able (a) to make better use of automated equipment because of work load concentration (b) to develop a wider range of specialised interests because of the ability given by staff concentration. This scheme has now been successfully operated for several years and the conclusion we draw is that a 400-600 bedded hospital with an Accident and Emergency Department, and Maternity Unit does not necessarily require all the pathology disciplines to be on site. Thus each discipline of pathology should make its own arrangements to cope with its own committments.

Such a scheme can only be operated if a good transport service has been developed together with adequate communications. At present we use the Rank Xerox telecopier, for result return and vans for specimen reception. The whole process has been easy to achieve because it is inside the barbed wire perimeter that constitutes the District boundary. This form of centralisation is common and has been known for years.

We will now consider an inter-District service in Chemical Pathology for the Hospitals shown in the diagram. In travelling time the furthest Hospital away from Hospital A is O which, as it is in the same district, receives its services from A. The other Hospitals however are to be found in four separate districts forming part of two different Areas. The problems have now ceased to be solely technical and include administrative and educational difficulties. There is a need to convince people that a different organisation of Clinical Chemistry may produce benefits, certainly if the level and sophistication of automation is increased. In addition, the range and depth of subjects in Clinical Chemistry which can be studied may be increased if the complex were considered as a whole.

To test whether an inter-district service was feasible an experiment was set us between the Districts centred on Hospitals

HW, A and S. These Hospitals are all close to a common railway line so the specimen transport system was based on British Rail; there are three trains per hour in each direction.

All electrolytes from the Districts centred on Hospital HW and Hospital S were analysed at Hospital A on a Technicon SMA 6/60. To check whether the service was degraded, as this mattered, all samples were duplicated and were analysed by the originating laboratory, in addition to the laboratory at Hospital A. Results were not sent out however, until those from Laboratory A were received back. All telephone calls for results were logged.

The electrolyte workload at A rose from 80 to 220, peaking at 300 on some days. The analytical system was stretched to its limit, which was one of the objects of the exercise. Figure 2 details the turn round times at Hospitals HW & S before the scheme, and illustrates the better level of service that HW could provide than S. During the scheme there was a considerable degradation of service at HW as Fig.3 shows. This was greater than at either S or A because the service at HW was initially better than either of the other two Hospitals were able to provide. Surprisingly very few telephone requests were received at S for results.

The conclusions we draw from the scheme are:
1. The SMA 6/60 was overloaded for much of the time and the stoppages which occurred due to blockages produced an unacceptable backlog of specimens.

2. The transport and telecopier system worked well.

3. If a faster machine had been available the outcome may have been different.

The series of estimations chosen was particularly sensitive and as facilities for these could not be withdrawn from S or HW the scheme was abandoned.

The introduction of an SMA 12/60 on which enzymes, Ca, P, Bilirubin, Albumin, Total Protein and Urate are determined reopened the whole question. Determination of these by a central laboratory was realised to be practical and has produced a conjoining of the laboratories at A & S for chemistry. There has been a complete reappraisal of where work is done and what should be done during extensive meetings of all the senior technical and graduate staff. These discussions have led to the creation of a radioimmunoassay service at S, a unit for major automation at A and agreement as to where a variety of other facets of chemistry should be developed, together with a rotation of staff to develop them.

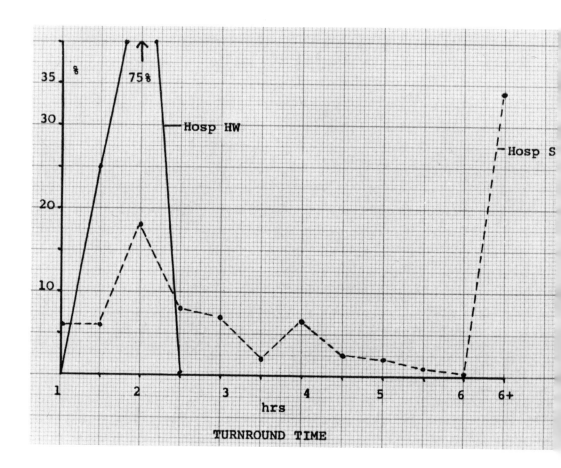

FIGURE 2

Turn round time of electrolytes, expressed as a percentage of the total load for hospitals HW and S before the electrolyte pilot study. Both hospitals had comparable systems for electrolytes (basically AAI methodology), HW (approximately 40 electrolytes per day) serves only one hospital with the majority of the work coming from in-patients, whilst S (approximately 100 electrolytes per day) serves two hospitals with a considerable amount of work coming from outpatient clinics.

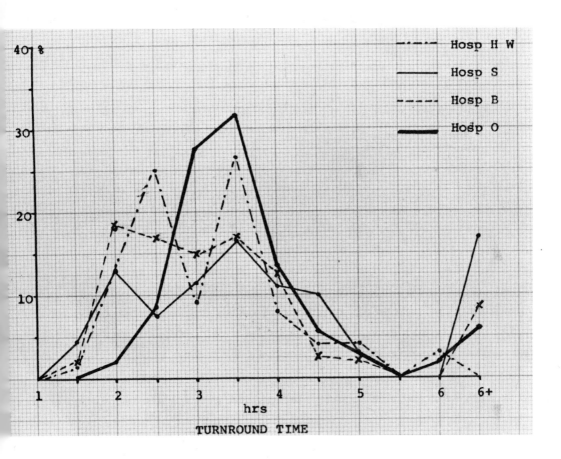

FIGURE 3

Turn round time of electrolytes expressed as a percentage of the total load for hospitals HW, S, B and O during the electrolyte pilot scheme. Note the increase turn round time of analyses for HW.

The scheme encompasses two Health Districts and has produced a large number of administrative complications. One suggestion is that the strategic administration should be at Area level so that the consequences of this conjoining on the rest of the Area can be evaluated and that a functional budget for the project should be produced. Probably functional administration should also occur at the same time, as the Physics service is linked in the same way. Of course other disciplines of Pathology may also wish to follow this development in their own way. If now, however, we hypothesize that instead of the SMA 12/60 we have more powerful analytical machinery in terms of speed and investigating range, then the potential work capacity is greater and it may be possible to contemplate the inclusion of other Districts into the scheme. The travelling distances are all feasible, but we now have the problem of developing a multi-district organisation. Possibly we should now be asking the fundamental question of, how many Clinical Chemistry Departments are required in a given geographical area to provide the service. Such a unit must be attractive for people to work in, and provide the clinician with results in a turn round time compatible with good medical practice.

Again the answers to questions such as this can only be given by experimentation and by not prejudging the results. We must not be frightened of possible change and must bear in mind that if we make trained manpower available we have created a more flexible situation. It is only by creating this degree of flexibility that we can start to argue, from a basis of experimentation, about the service we ought to be providing. It is only by creating this degree of flexibility that we can rapidly adjust to changing situations and new developments. Indeed we may hopefully start to create new developments. Centralisation as we see it is a means of providing such a degree of flexibility in addition to units which may investigate in depth, some facet of pathology. If centralisation is used for any other purpose, it will fail, because like any other rigid system it will not adapt, become unpleasant to work in and thus atrophy and die.

Discussion

Dr Wilding (Birmingham): Disciplines are pursuing independent paths in Pathology. Thus there is a lack of uniformity in the presentation of information to clinicians, and a loss in compatibility between haematology and clinical chemistry reports.

Dr Mills: In the area where the experiment was carried out, the hospitals were up to 6 miles apart and there was only a single discipline laboratory at each. However, between the separate laboratories there had been extensive discussion regarding the organisation of specimen collection and the style of report forms. Within the confines of the report form there is a general freedom in the manner in which data is reported. A computer would obviously require patient data for each discipline to be reported in a similar fashion, and this occurs already with our system.

Dr Buttolph (London): Most of the papers to be presented at this meeting have at least one feature in common: the implementation of the ideas expressed in them will require the spending of money, and this at a time when the prospects for NHS finance are not good. The present paper is different because it presents ideas which may result in financial savings.

At its inception, the NHS acquired a series of discrete laboratory units; the construction of an efficient, rationalised laboratory service is still far from complete. Although there are great differences in the amount of progress made in different parts of the country, many laboratories have been closed. Between 1963 and 1973, the number of clinical chemistry laboratories in England was reduced by one third. The closure of small units is worthwhile (because they are taken to be the least cost-effective) and relatively easy to accomplish (because the small amount of work undertaken can be absorbed by other laboratories). But the process cannot continue indefinitely and in due course it becomes necessary to undertake schemes which include larger units. Rationalisation of larger laboratories is most simply accomplished by providing a new building in which to carry out the work previously done at several separate sites. In the immediate future the capital needed for new building schemes will not be easily available. Thus in most cases, any rationalisation of laboratory services must be based on the accommodation already available. This constraint makes planning much more difficult, but the scheme that has been described demonstrates what can be accomplished without significant capital expenditure.

Dr Mills: Our primary objective was not solely one of saving money, but rather to look at the resources we had and see whether by re-distributing these we could provide ourselves with facilities in terms of staff, space and equipment for extending the range of investigations and thus possibly doing more interesting work. In addition, by drawing on a larger population we may now be able to justify setting up those assays which as individual districts neither of us could justify on economic grounds.

Dr Nicholson (London): What effect are the new administrative boundaries going to have on the rationalisation of laboratories, such as the closing of small, non-viable units? In particular, are there going to be any financial obstacles to sending specimens from one district, or even area, to another? One hopes that a broad-minded view will be taken.

Dr Mills: Within a district people tend to be very parochial. Thus administrators of a district tend to regard a single laboratory that serves two districts as having removed some financial resource from their district. Clinicians tend to regard a laboratory as their own, and the removal of this from a hospital is, in some way, seen as degrading the quality of the hospital and so it allegedly goes down in their estimation. If this attitude is admitted then the only way in which clinicians would be satisfied is to have all facilities duplicated in major individual hospitals, within a particular district, and the cost of this would be enormous.

KEEPING A BALANCE - SPECIALISED ANALYSES

W.H.P. Lewis

Regional Scientific Officer, S.E. Thames Regional
Health Authority
Randolph House, 46/48 Wellesley Road, Croydon, Surrey

Techniques available for the estimation of the levels of naturally occurring and administered compounds are becoming ever more complex. Such increases in the complexity of the reaction involved may result in the operator time increasing, or in the equipment required for carrying out the test being very sophisticated or indeed both. In some cases, however, relatively complex reaction sequences may be carried out simultaneously and rapidly and the operator involvement may be simplified. The costing of tests can be considered in terms of recurrent expenditure - staff, reagents etc. and non-recurrent apparatus.

Within the NHS there is normally separation between these two heads, and in fact, non-recurrent cost may be difficult to establish since the apparatus may be used for a number of different tests, for example, centrifuges or spectrophotometers. There are, however, a number of generalisations that may be made. For example, increasing the number of tests generally lowers the unit cost, but above the maximum batch size, the return is likely to be small. Conversely, small numbers of any particular test may be relatively expensive, and will, in any case, probably result in poor precision unless small batches are carried out frequently, so that the operator is familiar with the procedure.

The common solution to this problem is centralisation and the ultimate expression of this approach is the Supra Regional Laboratory Service established by the DHSS. The principle behind the Service is that certain laboratories, usually in Teaching Hospitals, have been designated as Supra-Regional Laboratories for particular assays, or more usually certain groups of assay, e.g. steroid hormones or tissue enzymes. In general, most of these laboratories are able to cope with the one-off assay from laboratories not normally carrying out the particular test, but they would be unable to cope with multiple tests from many different laboratories. It follows, therefore, that as the clinical requirement for a new test increases beyond a few tests in a given week for a particular hospital, it will need to be carried out at a more local level.

In the past, there has been a tendency for new tests to be established in an ad hoc manner, usually because a member of the staff of a particular hospital was interested in setting up a particular technique and the initiative may have come from clinical or laboratory staff. There is usually no particular incentive at the present time to evaluate the comparative cost of local versus centralised service for a particular test, since few laboratories work within a budget. Reagents are generally classified as drugs and as such little control is exercised within the District budget. However, one would expect that the accounting system within the NHS will change and that departmental budgets will become the rule rather than the exception. In these circumstances, therefore, it will be necessary for departmental managers to decide what the optimal allocation of their resources will be. The difficulty mainly lies in evaluating all the benefits of carrying out tests at local level, particularly on staff morale.

In recent years the cost per test in clinical chemistry at least, has been influenced by the introduction of multichannel analysers. With such machines it is cheaper to operate for twelve tests than older equipment for one, but there is a great tendency to calculate cost on the assumption that all tests are required. A reasonable average might be half the total, but once clinicians are aware of the capability of the equipment, they begin to request the whole profile since they know they will get all the results anyway.

Any attempt to make cost/benefit comparisons between tests will need to take into account a number of factors:

Cost of reagents and other disposable materials

Operator time

Equipment time - centrifuges, autoanalysers etc.

Clinical value, e.g. will patients' hospitalisation be affected
                 will diagnosis be simplified

Value of quick answer

Obviously not all of these factors can be quantified. It is, however, possible to calculate reagent and other costs, operator time, and therefore cost, without undue effort. It may also be possible, though rather more difficult to add a component for the

KEEPING A BALANCE — SPECIALISED ANALYSES

use of equipment. The other factors will be, in some degree at least, subjective.

The cost of consumables and labour will tend to fall as the number of tests carried out rises, but the steepness of the curve will tend to level off and a virtual plateau will be reached. The point at which the plateau is reached will depend upon a number of factors and will be different for autoanalytical techniques compared to manual. Autoanalysers needing long run up times like the Vickers MC300 or Technicon protein analyser, will need many more samples to reach economical levels than may be the case with manual techniques. On the other hand, given a high enough work load, they will usually compare very favourably with less sophisticated methods. Such equipment does, however, involve large capital investment which can be clearly identified with the test that it carries out, unlike the centrifuges and end point measuring equipment needed for manual methods.

At the other end of the scale, where relatively few tests of a particular type are done, there is an increasing tendency to use kits. Such kits may vary from a simple agar plate with a specific antibody included for the assay of a specific protein, to quite complex packs for radioimmunoassay or haemaglutination assay of hormones. Almost without exception, kits are relatively more expensive than in-house methods. Sometimes quality control leaves something to be desired, but there is little doubt that kits do enable the smaller laboratory to carry out assays which would otherwise be beyond their resources.

It would, however, be quite inappropriate to consider this area without at least attempting to look at the problem from the point of view of the consumer, that is, the patient and the tax payer. Availability of a service at local level may have a number of advantages for the patient - he may not need to travel so far, the test may speed diagnosis, his hospitalisation may be shorter, his treatment may begin earlier, other unnecessary tests and perhaps surgery may be avoided. All these points are also clearly to the advantage of the tax payer, but may be financially at least, outweighed if the cost per test is high, and will be quite invalidated if the precision is poor or unreliability results in repeat testing which may not only inconvenience the patient, but also unduly worry him.

It must be said, however, that the number of tests which can in themselves dramatically influence the course of a patient's treatment are in a minority and laboratory investigations simply form part of the whole spectrum of information available to the clinician. The complexity of non-clinical diagnostic information needed will clearly have to be related to the type of work carried out by the individual hospital, so that the presence of specialist units such as Renal Dialysis Units or Neurosurgical Units will very much influence the level of sophistication required and will again influence the balance of work. All too often, however, specialist units are established without considering what their effect on the workload of the service department will be, and it may well be a costly exercise to bring these departments up to the level required for an efficient service.

To take the above specific examples, a Neurosurgical Unit will require some very expensive x-ray equipment, preferably fairly close to the Operating Theatres, and a very rapid frozen section service. A Renal Dialysis Unit will generate many blood urea and electrolyte investigations, ideally carried out on minimum volumes of blood. There will be a requirement also for transfusion blood in the form of packed cells. Normally all patients admitted for dialysis will need testing for Australia Antigen. It is just possible that this could be sent out for testing with all likely dialysis patients tested as outpatients. From time to time, however, emergencies occur, and an anuric patient may need to be admitted. Failure to screen every patient would put all patients at risk. As it happens, the tests for Australia Antigen are not very complex but the safety precautions required are quite stringent for the protection of laboratory staff. We have therefore another constraint in the shape of the laboratory accommodation. Are there facilities for handling hazardous biological material, and if not, can space be provided to house them? All too frequently, the answer to both questions is no, with space being the overriding problem.

The final area which needs to be considered is the effect of the level of service on staff morale and training. There is clearly likely to be less satisfaction in working in a laboratory in which all the interesting work is sent out, than one in which there is a sophisticated repertoire of tests, provided that staff have the opportunity to move around. More importantly, junior staff need experience of a wide range of procedures if they are to be adequately trained and indeed this has now been recognised officially by the DHSS, who have,' for pathology, detailed which procedures should be available to staff in training grades.

The problems of maintaining a balance between routine and non-routine, simple and complex, inexpensive and expensive tests, can be seen to be a complex one. Inevitably some compromises will be necessary, given limited resources. The factors to be considered are the resources available, service to the patient, the effect on staff. Ultimately service to the patient should be the overriding consideration, but it must be remembered that unlimited resources are not available within the NHS, and they are unlikely to be within the foreseeable future. It is probably true to say that no NHS patient is denied any investigation which he needs, unless he is too ill to travel for an in vivo test. What we have to consider in practice is how best to utilise the resources at our disposal. The decisions will be difficult and sometimes unpopular with colleagues and patients. The introduction of a properly planned service should, however, mean that that best possible service is provided within the level of resources available.

LABORATORY DIAGNOSIS OF GENETIC PROBLEMS

L. J. Butler

Principal Cytogeneticist

Queen Elizabeth Hospital for Children
Hackney Road, London, E2 8PS

Classical Genetic Counselling

During the last twenty years, following the reduction of neonatal deaths and suffering from other (environmental) causes by antibiotic and immunization therapy, there has been a greater awareness of the genetically determined disorders and their contribution to congenital disease.

Accumulation of clinical data and, in some cases, the establishment of significant biochemical abnormalities has led to the delineation of progressively more genetic diseases. The total load of congenital disease is approximately 2% and the bulk of the problems are related in some way to the misfunction of the genes and there are nearly 2500 different conditions or syndromes now known which are wholly or partially genetically determined.

Gross changes of the chromosome pattern account for about 1% of all births, 9 out of every 10 showing some developmental abnormality. On the other hand, metabolic defects have an overall frequency of only about 1 per 1000 births which means that some enzyme defects are extremely rare.

The best known and most common single gene abnormality is the autosomal recessive mutant causing cystic fibrosis of the pancreas. The frequency at birth is about 1 in 2000 so that the gene frequency in the population is as high as 1 in 22.

The total number of individuals requiring genetic advice is therefore not numerous but, nevertheless, it would seem that perhaps one couple in 25 will need this advice urgently either because there are positive risks or simply for reassurance. The main reason for seeking advice in 85% of all cases is the birth of a child with some defect or other, and the remaining 15% are made up of those where a parent is already affected or there is something in the family history.

Genetic risks mostly fall into two categories either "good" with a recurrence of less than 1 in 20 or "bad" with a risk greater than 1 in 10. The latter are essentially abnormalities depending on either familial structural chromosome abnormalities or single gene defects, just over 50% of which have a dominant mode of inheritance (risk 1 : 2), nearly 40% autosomal recessive (risk 1 : 4) and about 8% X-linked recessive ($\frac{1}{2}$ males affected).

The "good" risk situations include all the common congenital malformations for example spina bifida, hare lip and congenital heart disease which are multifactorial in origin resulting from a complex interaction between several genes and the environment.

Accuracy of clinical diagnosis is extremely important especially with dominant conditions because of the sometimes variable manifestations. Parents must be examined carefully for minimal symptoms as for example in the condition tuberous sclerosis where one parent might show only a minor degree of adenoma sebaceum. The time of onset of disease is also important so that for conditions like Huntington's chorea which usually appears only in the middle thirties, the next generation at risk has already been produced. Dystrophia myotonica is variable in onset such that a child might develop the condition ahead of its also affected parent. Finally, accurate differentiation of similar conditions is very important as for example distinguishing between the severe dystrophic form of epidermiolysis bullosa from the simplex forms, the former being recessive and the latter dominant.

Heterozygote Detection : From a counselling point of view, it would be an obvious advantage if one could detect clinically normal heterozygotes of potentially lethal diseases, bearing in mind that the frequency of these carriers of single recessive mutants is much higher than the frequency of the disease (i.e. homozygotes). Although enzyme polymorphism and gene interactions can modify activities, in general it appears that gene dosage is very closely correlated with enzyme levels thus producing in the heterozygote with a single normal allele, a level halfway between the normal and the homozygous recessive.

Of course, in some conditions, the enzyme defect is only demonstrable in an inaccessible tissue such as the liver and, if measurements have to be restricted to the circulating or excreted metabolites, very often the levels between normals and heterozygotes overlap to such a degree that it is impossible to distinguish between them. Under these circumstances use is made of tolerance tests to stress the metabolic pathway in question. For example, in studies on phenylketonuria, the metabolism of a standard dose of phenylalanine, as measured by its disappearance from the plasma, is intermediate between normals and the affected homozygotes.

Other methods now exist for exaggerating the differences of activities in cells between normals, carriers and abnormals. Hirschhorn et al 1969 found that lymphocytes when transformed with PHA have a much higher α-glucosidase activity than the unaltered cells and, indeed, in heterozygotes for Pompe's disease, this enzyme remained constant. Nadler and Egen (1970) found the same kind of reaction in normals compared with carriers when investigating lysosomal acid phosphatase deficiency.

Increasing the level of the appropriate substrate for a particular enzyme in some instances, also increases the activity of that enzyme by a process known as gene derepression. We have used this for certain urea cycle enzymes especially the stimulation of argininosuccinic acid synthetase by adding citrulline to fibroblast cultures in investigation of citrullinaemia.

The detection of females heterozygous for X-linked recessive disorders is complicated by the process of X-inactivation (Lyon hypothesis) the net result of which is a mosaic effect for the enzyme defect. The best example is glucose-6-phosphate dehydrogenase deficiency (Beutler et al 1962) and the heterozygous state can be established by the histochemical demonstration of two cell populations either in red cells, hair root bulbs or cultured fibroblasts.

One problem of using cultured cells in which the population is essentially mixed in this way relates to the degree of metabolic co-operation which occurs between the cell types (Subak-Sharpe et al 1969). In the Lesch-Nyhan syndrome which is caused by a deficiency of the enzyme hypoxanthine-guanine phosphoribosyl transferase (HGPRT), the two populations of cells in fibroblast culture may be demonstrated by autoradiography (Rosenbloom et al. 1967) but the proportion of normal or HGPRT positive cells in cultures from heterozygotes tends to increase as the cell density increases (Dancis et al. 1969) thus complicating still further heterozygote detection.

Although good progress has been made in the detection of carriers of single mutant genes, the majority of metabolic abnormalities are so rare that population screening to detect the heterozygotes is out of the question so that even today, for the vast majority of conditions, the heterozygosity for the recessive disorder in the parents is only revealed for the first time by the appearance of their affected child.

Only small inbred populations with a high frequency of particular mutant genes (e.g. Tay Sachs and Gaucher's diseases in Ashkenazi Jews) are suitable for mass screening.

<u>The Value of Genetic Counselling - Feedback</u>: The value of genetic counselling can now be assessed from the follow-up studies which have been reported recently (Carter et al. 1971; Leonard et al. 1972 and Reynolds et al. 1974). Such retrospective analyses reveal important data on how far couples understood the information they were given, the decisions which they took regarding planning further pregnancies and, in some instances, a positive feedback from them as to how the counselling service could be improved.

In general, it was found that the parents had understood the information they were given and had, on the whole, taken responsible decisions on the basis of it. In the high risk category two-thirds were deterred from planning further children compared with only one quarter in the low risk group. The greater the severity of the handicap the more likely the parents were to be deterred. For example, in Carter's series (Carter et al. 1971) all 8 couples at risk of having a child with muscular dystrophy and 25 out of 29 couples where severe mental retardation was the problem were deterred. Comparable results from Leonard et al. 1972 are less favourable. They encountered rather different results when dealing with parents of families containing children with either cystic fibrosis, phenylketonuria or Down's syndrome and 25% appeared to have learned very little from the information given. There was in fact a higher percentage of patients from the lower socioeconomic classes in this series and, I quote, "many brought ignorance and sometimes hostility" to the consultation.

In view of this variability of response, there ought to be regional genetic registers to help follow up all members of such families at risk along the lines of the one established in Edinburgh by Emery (Smith et al. 1971) known as RAPID (Register for the Ascertainment and Prevention of Inherited Disease) or the FAMFL (Family File) system in operation in Oregon, U.S.A. (Kimberling, 1972).

A number of recommendations were made by those interviewed for improving genetic counselling. Most thought that there was a need for a wider distribution of information about the availability of genetic counselling services and several felt that they needed up to 6 months to adjust to the discovery of the birth defect or other genetic disease before being able to assimilate the counselling information. Many complained that they had not been informed of the need for extensive pedigree information to be available at the time of interview and some felt that insufficient explanation was given of the reason for laboratory tests, etc. Some would have appreciated a much longer interview session to allow them to talk more easily about their feelings and problems, and almost all welcomed the follow-up interview.

Obviously the whole problem is a complex one and, as such should be handled by a whole team of specialists including, paediatricians, obstetricians, medical geneticists, laboratory scientists, psychiatrists and social workers.

Fortunately recent developments in laboratory investigations are now transforming the whole field of genetic counselling and, for the diseases in question, we are able to speak of risks not in terms of 1 in 2 or 1 in 4 but of 0% or 100%! This very positive information is now obtainable before birth for an ever increasing range of disorders either by chemical investigations on the amniotic fluid or on the cytology and biochemical activities in the cells cultured from it.

Antenatal Diagnosis of Genetic Disorders

<u>Chromosomal Anomalies</u> : The starting point is a specimen of amniotic fluid which, for practical reasons, is collected at 15 - 16 weeks gestation by transabdominal amniocentesis. At this stage a reasonable cell population is present in the fluid and from an obstetric point of view, not only is it relatively much easier to collect especially with the use of ultrasound to locate the placenta, but virtually all natural abortions will have occurred before this time. Unfortunately amniocentesis is still not sufficiently safe for large scale use on low risk pregnancies as the abortion rate following the procedure seems to be about 1%.

The numbers of cells seen in the centrifuged specimen at first seems quite favourable (Fig. 1a) but only about 0.1% are capable of adhesion to the bottom of the culture vessel and then enter active cell division (Butler, 1972). The cells are derived from the surface of the amnion, the fetal epidermis and even the renal and respiratory epithelium (Butler and Reiss, 1970), and Fig. 1a shows a single ciliated cell (arrow) of this type closely adherent to a small group of non-ciliated epithelial cells.

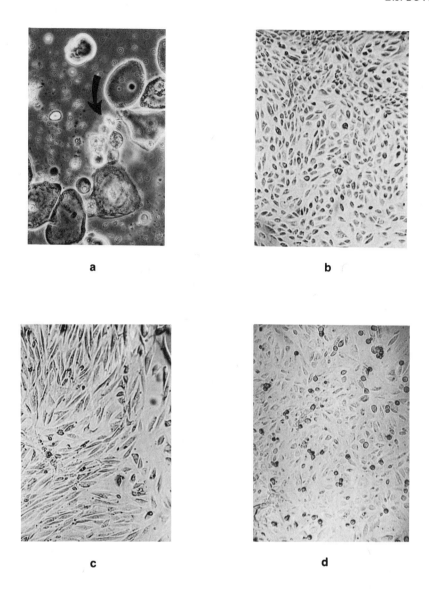

Fig. 1. Amniotic Fluid Cells: (a) Concentrated from a fresh sample of liquor (Note ciliated epithelial cell (arrow) referred to in text); (b-d) as seen in culture showing typical epithelial colony (b), fibroblastic growth (c) and extensive mitotic activity (= round dense cells) in an epithelial colony (d).

Most laboratories seem to have their own "recipe" for successful cell culture but the most commonly used media include either Medium 199 or Ham's F.10 in combination with fetal bovine serum at a concentration of 20% by volume (Butler, 1973). Not all batches of sera are entirely satisfactory; some have only modest growth potential whilst others are distinctly toxic. The latter can be improved sometimes by heat inactivation at 60°C for one hour whilst we have found that both can be supplemented with important growth factors contained in human cord serum added at the rate of only 2.5ml./100ml. serum. Since the introduction of cord serum our success rate for growth has increased from 95% with 1 in 20 of the amniocenteses having to be repeated to 100% with no repeats. Colonies of epithelial cells are present in virtually all culture vessels (Fig. 1b) but some contain fibroblasts (Fig. 1c) especially from specimens collected at 18 weeks or later. All cultures are particularly active mitotically after the 10th day in culture (Fig. 1d). Chromosome preparations are therefore obtained between the 10th and 20th day by direct growth of cells onto microscope slides (Butler et al. 1974) followed by automatic cytological processing and staining on a Shandon-Elliott machine (Fig. 2).

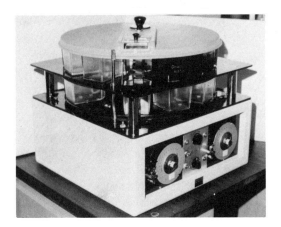

Fig. 2. Automatic Machine used for cytological processing (lower deck) and staining (upper deck).

TABLE 1. TOTAL ANTENATAL CHROMOSOME STUDIES PERFORMED IN THE WORLD > 3000

Screening for Down's Syndrome	% of Total		% Abnormal
(a) Familial	4.5)		22.0
(b) High Maternal Age	40.0)	80	3.0
(c) Previous regular trisomy	35.5)		1.5
Other Chromosome Anomalies			
(a) Familial	2.5)		16.0
(b) Previous trisomy	1.5)	20	0
(c) Other reasons	16.0)		0.5

Overall Abnormality Rate = 3.1%

Table 1 shows the percentage distribution of pregnancies studied so far based upon a world total of about 3,000 investigations. About 80% of all studies are aimed at the detection of Down's Syndrome (mongolism), regular trisomy 21, which is usually associated with high maternal age and is the most common sporadically occurring chromosome abnormality. The familial form, an unbalanced consequence of the segregation of a 14/21 translocation, is also one of the most frequently encountered structural alterations. Of course other numerical aberrations are also detected in screening the high maternal age group especially trisomies for Nos. 18 and 13 (Butler et al. 1973).

The new chromosome banding techniques (Pearson, 1972) are revealing even smaller structural alterations such as single band deletions (Fig. 3) and the investigations now required on each case are stretching the technical capacity to the limits. The fact that such additional studies are essential has been demonstrated in my own laboratory only recently with the discovery of a small de novo translocation between chromosomes Nos. 10 and 18 in the amniotic cells of the pregnancy of a woman aged 42. Children born with this type of anomaly are invariably mentally defective though their physical abnormalities may be slight. (This case will be reported in more detail elsewhere).

LABORATORY DIAGNOSIS OF GENETIC PROBLEMS 43

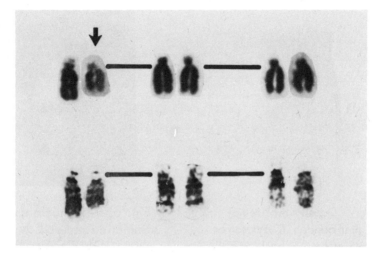

Fig. 3. Partial Karyotype (Group D) showing banded chromosomes (lower half) with a single band deletion in one of them (arrow).

The cell culture procedures and semi automated processing of chromosome material which we are using has reduced the handling time down to a minimum and to deal with even larger numbers of cases without having to increase the staff in proportion would require the introduction of automatic chromosome analysis on a large scale. Unfortunately the present day prototype pattern recognition systems which have been developed both in the U.S.A. and this country (Ledley and Ruddle, 1966; Rutovitz, 1968) are not particularly rapid and automatic cell selection presents special difficulties. Indeed, the human eye and brain together remain a much more efficient and discriminating combination. The instrumentation has been developed to trace the grey boundary between the edge of the chromosome and the background thus producing data on the relative length and position of the centromere. Now, of course, we need systems to take into account the recently discovered banding sequences along the length of the chromosomes. Density profiles (Fig. 4) can be obtained using instruments such as the Vickers M85 scanning microdensitometer which, suitably interfaced could be linked for automatic analysis. Given adequate computer facilities, a new version of such an instrument to scan the whole field rather than manual alignment for each chromosome, would represent a relatively inexpensive method of doing it. However, we must not forget that the banding makes it even easier for the human eye to cope efficiently.

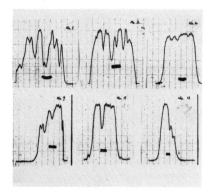

Fig. 4. Density profiles of individual banded chromosomes obtained using Vickers M85 Microdensitometer. Each peak represents a dense band.

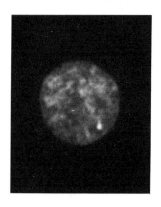

Fig. 5. The nucleus of an amniotic fluid cell showing the brightly fluorescent Y-body.

The pioneers in this aspect of automation are making good progress with the new style material (Lub and Ledley, 1973). The system developed by Castleman and Wall, 1973, which discriminates through 256 shades of grey offers the prospect of efficiency to match that of the retina, always providing of course that the chromosomes are well separated from each other. It is often not appreciated except by those working in the field that machines need perfect chromosome spreads on which to work whereas, in practice, the majority of cells produced, though good, are far from having this status. This is why automatic cell selection is such a hazardous business.

X-linked Genetic Disorders : Although establishment of the full karyotype based upon cell culture is desirable, the sex of the fetus can be determined on the same day as the fluid is collected by staining preparations of fixed cells from the suspension. Vital dyes are used to reveal the X-chromatin body in the nuclei when two X chromosomes are present, and similar preparations are treated with fluorescent compounds of the quinacrine group to demonstrate the Y-body (Fig. 5). This staining combination gives a reliability for sex determination of $> 99\%$ to permit an early termination of pregnancy when a male fetus is present. Indeed, abnormal sex chromosome complements have already been predicted before the full karyotype was obtained by finding nuclei which were positive for both X and Y bodies i.e. a male fetus with XXY. (Walker et al. 1971). Fetal sex determination is widely used in the management of pregnancies where Duchenne muscular dystrophy and haemophilia are inherited problems.

Metabolic Disorders: The range of metabolic abnormalities which can now be detected by the demonstration of a specific enzyme deficiency in the cultured amniotic fluid cells, can be appreciated from Table 2. The asterisk indicates those conditions which have been studied by at least one laboratory in the U.K. and the Clinical Genetics Society is keeping an up-to-date register. The storage diseases involving abnormal metabolism of glycogen and lipid and the mucopolysaccharidoses are the most widely investigated so far, especially Tay Sachs disease. The prospects for accurate diagnosis are enhanced not only by specific enzyme estimations but also by demonstration of the storage biproducts caused by the enzyme deficiency within the cells.

The main problems are related to the activities of enzyme systems in cultured cells. Some enzymes are either not required in their metabolism when growing as monolayers, the code for their production is switched off, or the levels are extremely low in normal cells. Broadly speaking the enzyme complements of epithelial cells and fibroblasts are similar with the exception of histidase and cystathionine synthetase activities, epithelial cells having a higher level of the former whilst fibroblasts have a higher level of the latter. (Gerbie et al. 1972). The cell types used in the investigation of histidinaemia and homocystinuria are therefore very important.

Time for this paper does not permit a more detailed appraisal of these disorders except to emphasize that there is no question of screening random low risk pregnancies. In view of the time required to produce sufficient cultured cells for a single enzyme assay, it is only possible to screen the pregnancies in known high risk families. As the overall frequency of metabolic disease at birth is only about 0.1% a mass screening programme is hardly justified. For rapid results one could only produce biochemical profiles of the amniotic fluid which does not show dramatic departures in its constitution even when the fetus is abnormal except for the major CNS defects referred to later. Therefore identification and elimination of the fetus with a biochemical abnormality in known families will make only a very small impact on the reduction of the numbers of such retarded individuals. Furthermore as these families will be less inhibited about having children in the future, the number of heterozygous carriers of the diseases will increase because only homozygous fetuses will be aborted.

TABLE 2   ANTENATAL DIAGNOSIS OF METABOLIC DISORDERS

Disorders of Carbohydrate Metabolism

Disease	Accumulated Products	Enzyme Deficiency
* FUCOSIDOSIS	Fucose containing hetero-polysaccharide	α-Fucosidase
* GALACTOKINASE DEFICIENCY	Galactose	Galactokinase
* GALACTOSAEMIA	Galactose	Galactose-1-P-uridyl transferase
GLUCOSE-6-PHOSPHATE DEHYDROGENASE DEFICIENCY		G-6-P-D
* GLYCOGEN STORAGE		
Pompe's - Type II	Glycogen Storage	α-1, 4-Glucosidase
Forbes - Type III	Abnormal Glycogen	Amylo-1,6-Glucosidase
Anderson's - Type IV	Abnormal Glycogen	α-glucan branching glycosyl transferase
Her's - Type VI	Abnormal Glycogen	Glycogen phosphorylase
MANNOSIDOSIS	Mannose and Glucosamine containing hetero-polysaccharide	α-Mannosidase
PYRUVATE DECARBOXYLASE DEFICIENCY	Pyruvic Acid, Alanine and Lactate	Pyruvate Decarboxylase

Disorders of Lipid Metabolism

Disease	Accumulated Products	Enzyme Deficiency
FABRY'S	Ceramidetrihexoside	Ceramidetrihexoside α-Galactosidase
* G_{M1} GANGLIOSIDOSIS Generalised Gangliosidosis - Type I Juvenile - Type II	G_{M1} Ganglioside and Ceramide Tetrahexoside	β-Galactosidase A, B and C
* G_{M2} GANGLIOSIDOSIS Tay Sachs - Type I Sandhoff's - Type II	G_{M2} Ganglioside and its Asialo Derivative	N-acetyl Hexosaminidase Hexosaminidase A and B
* GAUCHER'S	Glucocerebroside	β-Glucocerebrosidase
* KRABBE'S Globoid cell leucodystrophy	Galactocerebroside	Galactocerebroside β-Galactosidase
* METACHROMATIC LEUKODYSTROPHY	Sulphatide	Arylsulphatase A (Sulphatidase)
NIEMANN-PICK	Sphingomyelin	Sphingomyelinase
REFSUM'S	Phytanic Acid	Phytanic Acid Oxidase
* WOLMAN'S		Acid lipase esterase

LABORATORY DIAGNOSIS OF GENETIC PROBLEMS 47

TABLE 2 (Cont'd.)

Disorders of Amino Acid Metabolism

Disease	Accumulated Products	Enzyme Deficiency
*MAPLE SYRUP URINE (Severe Infantile)	Valine, Leucine, Isoleucine, Alloiso-leucine	Branched Chain Keto Acid Decarboxylase
HYPERVALINAEMIA	Valine	Valine Transaminase
*METHYLMALONIC ACIDAEMIA	Methylmalonic Acid, Glycine, Homocystine & Cystathionine	Methylmalonic CoA isomerase or Vit B_{12} coenzyme
*PROPRIONICACIDAEMIA	Glycine	Proprionyl CoA Carboxylase
HOMOCYSTINURIA	Methionine and Homocystine	Cystathionine Synthetase
CYSTATHIONINURIA	Cystathionine	Homoserine dehydratase
ARGININOSUCCINIC ACIDURIA	Argininosuccinic Acid	Argininosuccinase
CITRULLINAEMIA	Citrulline	Argininosuccinic Acid Synthetase
HYPERAMMONAEMIA	Ammonia → Glutamine	Ornithine Transcarbamylase
ORNITHINE - α-KETOACID TRANSAMINASE DEFICIENCY	Ornithine	Ornithine - α-Ketoacid Transaminase
HYPERARGININAEMIA	Arginine	Arginase
HISTIDINAEMIA	Histidine	Histidine α-deaminase
HYPERLYSINAEMIA	Lysine	Lysine-ketoglutarate Reductase
*CYSTINOSIS	Cystine	Unknown

Miscellaneous Metabolic Disorders

Disease	Enzyme Deficiency
ACATALASAEMIA	Catalase
ADRENOGENITAL SYNDROME	Failure of C21, C11 or steroid hydroxylation
CHEDIAK-HIGASHI SYNDROME	Unknown
ERYTHROPOIETIC PORPHYRIA	Co synthetase
HYPOPHOSPHATASIA	Alkaline phosphatase
I-CELL DISEASE	(β-glucuronidase reduced (Acid phosphatase raised
LACTOSYL CERAMIDOSIS	Lactosyl ceramide β-galactosidase
LESCH-NYHAN SYNDROME	Hypoxanthine - guanine - phosphoribosyl - transferase
LYSOMAL ACID PHOSPHATASE DEFICIENCY	Acid phosphatase
OROTIC ACIDURIA	Orofidylic pyrophosphorylase and decarboxylase
XERODERMA PIGMENTOSUM	DNA "repair" enzyme.

TABLE 2 (Cont'd.)

The Mucopolysaccharidoses

Disease	Enzyme Deficiency
* HURLER'S SYNDROME - Type I	α-1-iduronidase
* HUNTER'S SYNDROME - Type II	Sulphoiduronate sulphatase
* SANFILIPPO SYNDROME Type III	(Heparan sulphamidase (A) (- acetyl hexosaminidase (B)
MORQUIO'S SYNDROME - Type IV	Unknown
SCHEIE'S SYNDROME - Type V	α-1-iduronidase
MAROTEAUX - LAMY SYNDROME - Type VI	Unknown

Spina Bifida and Anencephaly: In 1972, Brock and Sutcliffe, using an electrophoresis method for protein separation, discovered that the level of alpha$_1$ - fetoprotein (α-FP) in the amniotic fluid is significantly raised when the fetus has a major defect of the central nervous system i.e. open spina bifida and/or anencephaly. Collectively these are very common congenital malformations with a birth frequency of 1 per 200 and, as genetic components have a role in the aetiology, the risk for subsequent pregnancies is increased (= about 1 in 25). For the time being pregnancies at special risk are being studied but with the introduction of the radio immunoassay method of Ruoslahti and Seppala (1971), mass screening has become possible. It is now known that the maternal serum levels of α-FP are also raised when the fetus is defective (Leek et al. 1973). Although about 1% of serum samples can give a falsely elevated level, with further refinement of assay method, amniocentesis should only be necessary in 2 or 3% of all cases.

Therefore by routinely estimating the α-FP and producing the karyotype from cultured cells on every amniotic fluid collected we are screening for the two most common congenital malformations viz. Down's Syndrome and spina bifida. The value of double screening is demonstrated by our recent discovery of CNS defects in two fetuses where the risk of Down's Syndrome was the main cause for concern.

LABORATORY DIAGNOSIS OF GENETIC PROBLEMS

TABLE 3.   INDICATIONS FOR ANTENATAL DIAGNOSIS

A   RISK > 1 in 20

1. Familial chromosome translocation
2. X-linked recessive disorders
3. X-linked dominant or autosomal recessive disorders lethal to males
4. Autosomal recessive disorders (mainly metabolic)
5. Autosomal dominant disorders (e.g. inherited myotonic dystrophy by linkage studies)

B   RISK between 1 in 20 and 1 in 100

1. Random chromosome abnormalities especially Down's Syndrome at maternal age > 35 or following previous regular trisomy.
2. Certain congenital malformations e.g. CNS defects by α-fetoprotein studies, hare-lip and polydactyly by fetoscopy.

Summary and Conclusions: The new developments which I have briefly outlined are clearly a major step forward in the management of genetically based diseases but there are a number of problems still awaiting solution and some aspects where technique needs to be improved. I have recently carried out a critical analysis of all phases of the art (Butler, 1973) - an art which Steele (1973) regards as being "far removed from the cook book stage required for broad applicability". In addition we do not yet know what the overall effects are on the normal fetus subjected to the slight traumas of amniocentesis and ultrasound at this early stage of pregnancy.

We must therefore apply these investigations wisely and consider for the time being only the categories as listed in Table 3 where the risk exceeds 1 in 100. After a further 5 years of detailed analysis we should have sufficient data concerning risks to both mother and fetus and may be the resources as well to safely screen pregnancies on a larger scale.

Acknowledgement: I would like to thank Miss I.K. Haverly for typing the manuscript.

BEUTLER, E, YEH, M. and FAIRBANKS, V.F. (1962),
Proc. Natn. Acad. Sci., U.S.A. $\underline{48}$, 9.

BROCK, D.J.H. and SUTCLIFFE, R.G. (1972), Lancet $\underline{II}$, 197.

BUTLER, L.J. and REISS, H.E. (1970)
J. Obstet. Gynaec. Brit. Cwlth. $\underline{77}$, 902.

BUTLER, L.J. (1972) in "Mental Retardation: Prenatal Diagnosis and Infant Assessment." Ed. Douglas, C.P. and Holt, K.S. pp. 1-16
(Butterworth, London).

BUTLER, L.J. (1973) "Antenatal Chromosome Studies: Current Problems" in Proceedings of 3rd International Congress IASSMD, The Hague, September, 1973. Ed. Primrose, D.A.A. pp. 573-578.

BUTLER, L.J., REISS, H.E., FRANCE, N.E. and BRIDDON, S. (1973), J. Med. Genet. $\underline{10}$, 367.

BUTLER, L.J., BRIDDON, S. and JACKSON, E.L. (1974). Humangenetik, $\underline{22}$, 229.

CARTER, C.O., FRASER ROBERTS, J.A., EVANS, K.A. and BUCK, A.R. (1971), Lancet $\underline{I}$, 281.

CASTLEMAN, K.R. and WALL, R.J. (1973) in "Chromosome Identification technique and applications in biology and medicine" Ed. Caspersson, T. and Zeck, L. Proceedings 23rd Nobel Symposium, Academic Press, pp. 77-84.

DANCIS, J., COX, R.P., BERMAN, P.H., JANSEN, V. and BALIS, M.E. (1969), Biochem. Genet. $\underline{3}$, 609.

GERBIE, A.B., MELANCON, S.B., RYAN, C. and NADLER, H.L. (1972), Amer. J. Obstet. Gynec. $\underline{114}$, 314.

HIRSCHHORN, K., NADLER, H.L., WAITHE, W.T., BROWN, B.I. and HIRSCHHORN, R. (1969), Science, $\underline{166}$, 1632.

KIMBERLING, W.J. (1972) in "Perspectives in Cytogenetics. The next decade" Edited by Wright, S.W., Crandall, B.F. and Boyer, L. Springfield, Illinois, Charles C. Thomas, Pub. pp. 131-147.

LEDLEY, R.S. and RUDDLE, F.H. (1966), Sci. Amer. 214, 40.

LEEK, A.E., RUOSS, C.F., KITAU, M.J. and CHARD, T. (1973), Lancet II, 385.

LEONARD, C.O., CHASE, G.A. and CHILDS, B. (1972), New Eng. J. Med. 287, 433.

LUBS, H.A. and LEDLEY, R.S. (1973) in "Chromosome Identification technique and applications in biology and medicine" Ed. Caspersson, T. and Zeck, L. Proceedings 23rd Nobel Symposium, Academic Press, pp. 61-76.

NADLER, H.L. and EGAN, T.J. (1970), New Eng. J. Med. 282, 596.

PEARSON, P. (1972), J. Med. Genet. 9, 264.

REYNOLDS, B. DeV., PUCK, M.H. and ROBINSON, A. (1974), Clin. Genet. 5, 177.

ROSENBLOOM, F.M., KELLY, W.N., HENDERSON, J.F. and SEEGMILLER, J.E. (1967), Lancet II, 305

RUOSLAHTI, E. and SEPPALA, M. (1971). Int. J. Cancer, 8, 374.

RUTOVITZ, D. (1968), Brit. med. Bull. 24, 260.

SMITH, C., HOLLOWAY, S. and EMERY, A.E.H. (1971), J. Med. Genet. 8, 453.

STEELE, M.W. (1973), Lancet, I, 542.

SUBAK-SHARPE, H., BURK, R.R. and PITTS, J.D. (1969), J. Cell Sci. 4, 353.

WALKER, S., GREGSON, N.M. and HIBBARD, B.M. (1971), Lancet, II, 430

Discussion

Dr Wilding (Birmingham) questioned whether the present state of technology and facilities available justified the use of these tests for screening pregnancies at lower risk, pointing out that there were still large differences in success rates between laboratories.

Mr Butler agreed that it would be undesirable for laboratories with only a limited experience of cell culture techniques to attempt these new procedures and he emphasised that he was against the proliferation of small cytogenetic units in ordinary general hospitals. These services should be organised on a regional basis with one designated laboratory having long experience being responsible for the culture of the amniotic fluid cells. His own experience in the NE Thames Region had demonstrated that the appropriate co-operation between the consultant obstetricians, either directly or via the pathologists, can be achieved without too much difficulty.

Interlaboratory co-operation on a national scale is clearly essential when dealing with many of the metabolic problems for, as these are individually rare, the expertise for particular assays is concentrated in one or two centres only. Restriction of antenatal studies to regional centres should help to curb a tendency for some laboratories to attempt investigations of this kind which are too limited and spread so thinly that they become worthless.

Regarding the relative cost of these investigations, the speaker agreed with a comment made earlier from the floor that laboratory studies in genetics were expensive but he pointed out that for a relatively small investment money was being saved in the long term as a result of introducing antenatal screening. Given the abnormality rates already established, every fetus aborted who would have survived its first year of post-natal life to become developmentally abnormal and who would thus have required either institutionalization or other social service support had it not been identified, represented a net saving to the nation of at least £15 000.

DISCUSSION

<u>Dr Taylor</u> (Toronto) strongly supported the view expressed by the speaker and hoped that there would be further expansion in this important aspect of preventative medicine. He mentioned that there were many factors to be considered other than purely financial ones.

PART II

Radiation Diagnostics

PROVISION OF A MAMMOGRAPHY SERVICE

M. Davison

Department of Clinical Physics and Bio-Engineering
West of Scotland Health Boards, 11 West Graham Street
Glasgow, G4 9LF

Breast cancer is the commonest cause of death from malignant disease in women. Statistics indicate 1 in 17 women develop it in some form or other, and it is responsible for nearly 10,000 deaths per year in the U.K. In view of these figures it is very hard to understand why there has been such a lack of interest by Radiologists in possible diagnostic techniques. The five year survival figures have hardly changed over the last thirty years despite advances in surgery and radiotherapy. This may well be because the disease has reached a late stage before the patient becomes aware of it. Although self-examination of the breast has been recommended the indications are that tumour diameters approach 3.5 cm before discovery, and by that time 65% of them are no longer localised. The prognosis should be improved the smaller the tumour and the earlier in its development it is discovered. Although there is no real evidence for this supposition it does seem reasonable to expect that the earlier the diagnosis is made the easier it is to institute effective treatment. This might in some cases mean less mutilating surgery.

Surveys have shown that early diagnosis can be achieved by both clinical examination and by the radiographic technique of Mammography, the detected tumours being both smaller and associated with a lower incidence of axillary node metastases. Detection efficiencies of 90% can now be obtained with each technique separately and can approach 100% when the techniques are used in complement, since the clinical examination is more effective with the highly glandular breast and mammography is better at detecting small tumours in the large fatty breasts.

RADIOGRAPHIC APPEARANCE

Consider first of all the normal breast. The adolescent breast consists mainly of dense granular tissue. Radiographs tend to be of poor quality and very little detail is visible in the gland structure, which appears as a fan-shaped homogeneous mass extending from the nipple. In the adult glandular breast fatty infiltration and fibrous ligaments create confusing patterns. With age the gland becomes progressively replaced by fat and hence becomes more radiolucent so that tumours are more readily observed. The effect of pregnancy, lactation or the pill is to cause physiological changes leading to a massive increase in glandular shadow making the detection of small isolated carcinomas more difficult.

The mammographic technique relies on the fact that breast tumours are slightly denser than normal tissue, and have well defined structures. To enhance the low X-ray contrast the technique is to use as low a kilovoltage and filtration as possible. The lower the kilovoltage the smaller the tumour that can be seen, the practical limit being of the order 5 mm. At the same time the skin dose to the patient will increase. The presence of minute specks of calcification, a fraction of a millimetre in diameter, occurring within the tumour is an additional feature that considerably helps diagnosis. It occurs in 40% of proven cases, and to adequately record these it is necessary to use an X-ray tube with a fine focal spot. Skin thickening and vessel asymmetry are other features that may well be present and help confirm the diagnosis.

TYPE OF X-RAY TUBE

The requirement of low kilovoltage and fine focal spot is difficult to satisfy with conventional tungsten anode X-ray tubes. Kilovoltages below 40 can not normally be used because the low radiation output would lead to excessive exposure times. However, molybdenum anode tubes recently developed give rise to adequate radiation outputs at 18 kilovolts and this probably represents the optimum compromise between contrast and patient skin dose. The radiation from such a tube, when filtered by molybdenum rather than aluminium, is concentrated into the K-characteristic radiation, which conveniently corresponds in energy to the maximum sensitivity of the photographic emulsion. The effect of increasing the kilovoltage across the X-ray tube is to increase the output without any significant change in the energy so that the radiation contrast in the image is unchanged. Operation at 35 KV is typically used.

TECHNIQUE

Two views are normally taken of each breast, one cranio-

PROVISION OF A MAMMOGRAPHY SERVICE

caudal and one lateral. Special shaped cones are used to limit the radiation to the breast alone, and give compression to fix the breast and to minimise the tissue thickness to be penetrated. Reduction of the irradiated volume decreases scatter and improves the contrast. It is necessary to obtain as much detail as possible through the whole breast including those tissues close to the ribs. This requires a beam projection running tangentially to the thoracic wall, which cannot easily be achieved with the conventional design of tube, and so purpose built units have the focus of the tube, the front edge of the cone and the edge of the film all in line. The patient is normally seated. The X-ray tube and film support are coupled together and can be easily manoeuvred into the required projections.

Even following compression the inner portions of the breast will absorb X-rays very much more than the peripheral skin areas. A film of high latitude is therefore required, giving a wide range of densities on the film. A non-screen industrial type capable of recording the fine calcifications is normally used, and because the film contrast increases with density then an average optical density of 2 is used instead of the value 1 more normal in general medical radiography. Viewing of the film can then be quite a problem, since it is not easy to pick out details in both the light areas of the chest wall and in the very dense areas round the nipple. Good masking with a variable intensity light box is essential to be certain of appreciating all the recorded information. The whole technique is by no means simple and requires great care throughout.

IMAGE ENHANCEMENT

When considering the contrast threshold of detection it should be realised that the eye recognises most objects by virtue of boundaries rather than absolute light levels. The sharper the edge the more readily the object is recognised. Significant improvements in detection could be made if it were possible to enhance the border effect. This can be done for example by viewing a conventional film with a television processing unit that suppresses the low spatial frequencies, or by copying with the Logetronic process. The recent introduction of Xero radiography gives the possibility of producing enhanced radiographs directly, and this technique has been found very suitable for mammograms. In the Xerox process a re-usable selenium plate is exposed to the radiation and the image is produced as a paper copy in either the positive or the negative mode. The blood vessels, ducts, skin and tumour edges are all well defined and stand out clearly.

Comparisons made between conventional films and Xero radiographs show that not only is the Xerox superior to the film in visualising small particles such as calcifications, but by virtue of its low overall contrast it is able to delineate the whole of the breast from the chest wall to the skin surface in one image. These superior results in fact can be obtained with a conventional tungsten X-ray tube giving a lower radiation dose to the patient than a molybdenum tube, the skin dose in this case being of the order 4 rad per exposure.

IS IT A SCREENING PROCEDURE?

The purpose of mammography can be summarised as
1) Early detection.
2) Differential diagnosis.
3) Localisation of the tumour.

As mentioned earlier the tumour detection rate when combined with a clinical examination can approach 100% so that the false positive and false negative rates can be neglected. In the ideal case malignant growths can be distinguished from benign on the mammogram. Benign masses tend to be homogeneously dense, with a rounded or smoothly lobulated border, and they push the normal tissues aside. The malignant tumours because of their more active growth have a denser centre and irregular spiculated borders invading the surrounding tissues, and normally are associated with skin thickening. But it is not always possible to distinguish between benign and malignant growths. In equivocal cases the examination can be repeated after a time interval, or biopsy samples can be taken using the radiographs as a guide to direction and position. Of course to achieve high accuracy of diagnosis great care must be put into all aspects of the technique - the radiation quality, exposure, processing and viewing.

In spite of these limitations its use as a routine screening procedure must be considered. If we consider the age incidence of breast cancer we can identify the 35 to 55 year age group as requiring special attention, because of the social implications of this age group involved with family responsibilities. This would give something over 8M examinations per year in England and Wales, and if we compare this with a figure of about 15M X-Ray investigations currently carried out we realise that a considerable effort and expense would be involved in this additional commitment. The expected incidence and detection rate is of the order 1 to 2 per thousand for this age group and in terms of cost effectiveness this begins to look a very poor return on investment. For an earlier age group the incidence is much less than 1 per thousand and although it rises higher for older age groups this increase is more than offset by the rising incidence of other causes of death. Screening can only be justified, if at all, for the age group 35 to 55.

The hazard of carrying out a screening survey has to be considered, in view of the possibility of causing radiation induced cancer while trying to detect it. Tumours have been reported following excessive chest fluoroscopy and radiotherapy. The risk however at 2 rad/breast/annum is considered negligible. So that current developments are aimed at finding a satisfactory combination of film and screen to give adequate quality with a lower dose than is required for non screen film or Xerographic plates. Using a single screen in a simple vacuum pack to get optimum film screen contact promising results have been achieved with a dose as low as 0.3 R.

No doubt technical developments will continue, but the problem now seems to be more political. Can the Health Service afford to screen the 8M women at risk? Or is the technique better restricted to certain high risk groups such as those who have already had mastectomy, those with a family history of the disease or symptoms of persistent breast pain. The problem then becomes not one of cost but to improve diagnostic accuracy and reduce the number of equivocal cases, and this requires great experience on the part of the Radiologists.

This paper is based on work carried out in conjunction with Dr. W.B. James and Dr. A.L. Evans (in the Department of Radiology) at the Southern General Hospital, Glasgow.

ULTRASONIC DIAGNOSTICS : CAPABILITIES OF PRESENT SYSTEMS

P. N. T. Wells

Bristol General Hospital

Bristol BS1 6SY, U.K.

ABSTRACT

No matter what the final display may be, similar considerations apply to the resolutions of all ultrasonic pulse-echo systems. In range, the resolution is determined by the duration of the pulse, and in azimuth and elevation, by the width of the beam. The pulse is generally the limiting component, and the dimensions of the scanned anatomy control the choice of wavelength. Gray scale display of a wide range of echo amplitude can give additional diagnostic information. In Doppler systems, zero-crossing detectors can give rise to errors, which can largely be avoided by the use of frequency spectrum analysis.

PULSE-ECHO SYSTEMS: RESOLUTION AND DISPLAY

All ultrasonic pulse-echo systems are based on the same physical principles [1]. When a pulse of ultrasound is transmitted into a body, it travels through the soft tissues at a velocity of about 1 500 m s^{-1}. A proportion of the energy is reflected or scattered at interfaces where there is a change in characteristic impedance. The characteristic impedance of a material is the product of its density and the velocity of ultrasound within it. Pulse-echo diagnostics depend on the measurement of the times of arrival of these echoes, which depend on the distances along the ultrasonic beam of the corresponding reflecting surfaces, and on the measurement of the amplitudes of the echoes, which depend on many factors including characteristic impedance, size, and attenuation.

Pulse-echo data may be displayed or analysed in many different ways. The most usual displays are the A-scope where time, and hence distance, is shown on one axis of a graph, usually on a cathode ray tube, and the occurrence of echoes is shown on the other axis — and the two dimensional B-scope, in which a scanning instrument allows a plane to be scanned, and the display is brightness-modulated and integrated to form a two-dimensional image of the corresponding section across the patient.

No matter what the final display may be, similar considerations apply to the resolutions of all ultrasonic pulse-echo systems. The resolution is equal to the minimum distance between two point targets at which separate registrations can just be distinguished on the display. An alternative definition is to specify the distance on the display which appears to be occupied by a point target in the field. This second definition, which is equivalent in concept to the first, is more convenient to implement in practice, and avoids difficulties due to interference between the echoes from two targets.

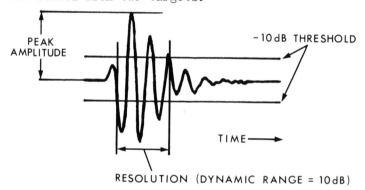

Fig. 1. Pulse response of a typical diagnostic ultrasonic probe. The −10 dB threshold level is indicated, together with the resolution for the corresponding dynamic range.

The range resolution depends on the shape of the ultrasonic echo, and the characteristics of the receiver. In any system, it is the transducer which is generally the component which has the greatest influence on the echo shape. The waveform of a typical echo pulse at the output from the transducer is illustrated in Fig. 1. Whatever signal processing may be applied to the pulse in the receiver, there is some threshold level which the input amplitude needs to exceed in order to produce a registration on the display. For the purpose of estimating the resolution the duration of the echo may be taken to be equal to the time for which the echo envelope exceeds this threshold. The resolution is equal to the distance in the medium corresponding to this time interval (approximately 0.75 mm μs^{-1}), increased by a distance depending on the bandwidth of the receiver electronics, and by a distance corresponding to the spot size of the display. Other things being equal, the resolution is proportional to the duration of the pulse, and this depends on four main factors. These are the form of electrical excitation (usually a unidirectional transient of short duration), the resonance frequency of the transducer, the bandwidth of the probe, and the attenuation of the ultrasonic propagation path (which acts as a low-pass filter). The 10 dB bandwidth of the overall transfer function of a pulse-echo probe is typically 50% of the resonance frequency [2], and so the resolution is approximately proportional to the wavelength of the ultrasound. In general, a typical system has range resolutions of about 1.0, 1.7 and 2.2 wavelengths with dynamic ranges of 10, 20 and 30 dB respectively [1]. The wavelength is about 1 mm at a frequency of 1.5 MHz. In principle, the range resolution may be improved by the use of higher frequency, but in practice the frequency is limited by absorption. In biological soft tissues, the swept gain rate required to compensate for absorption is about 1.3 N dB cm^{-1}, where N is the nominal value of the frequency measured in megahertz[1]. This corresponds to about 0.20 dB per wavelength. Within the limitations imposed by noise and by the maximum transmitted power, the maximum dynamic range of the echoes received in medical diagnostic pulse-echo systems is about 100 dB [3]. Of this, 30 dB might be required for variations in target strength — although, as discussed later, this would correspond to a poor lateral resolution — and so 70 dB might be available for swept gain. This corresponds to a maximum penetration of 350 wavelengths. Unfortunately, errors in swept gain compensation — due to uncertainties in attenuation rates — make it necessary to use a higher than optimum system gain, and in conventional systems it is unusual for the swept gain range to exceed 40 dB, or 200 wavelengths. In any particular clinical application, the distance which must contain these 200 wavelengths is determined by the scale of the scanned anatomy.

The lateral resolution — the resolution in azimuth or in elevation — is equal to the effective diameter of the ultrasonic beam. Typical beam profiles for a plane transducer are illustrated in Fig. 2. The transducer diameter is 20 wavelengths, and at a range of 100 wavelengths, the resolutions are 10, 16 and 25 wavelengths with dynamic ranges of 10, 20 and 30 dB respectively. Most modern ultrasonic pulse-echo instruments use weakly-focused transducers [4], and typically, in relation to a plane transducer of the same diameter, the lateral resolution may be improved by a factor of about two at a range of 100 wavelengths, whilst being similar at ranges of 0 and 200 wavelengths, but worse at greater ranges.

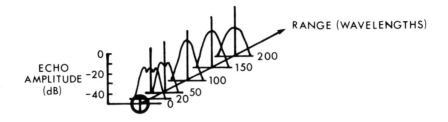

Fig. 2. Beam profiles for a pulse-echo transducer of 20 wavelengths diameter [1].

In the absence of focusing, the lateral resolution is about ten times worse then the range resolution. The resolution cell, which is the volume of tissue within which the interaction providing the diagnostic data takes place, is, to a first approximation, an ellipsoid with its short axis coincident with the central axis of the ultrasonic beam.

This discussion of resolution has taken into account the dynamic range of the signals which are displayed by the system, and it is implicit that this dynamic range is compressed to zero at the display. This condition would normally not be satisfied with an A-scope, in which the display dynamic range is around 40 dB, although it would be with a B-scope either if a bistable storage tube is used, or with certain signal processing schemes, or with high-contrast photography. Indeed, in some instruments, the signal is processed so that a pulse of defined amplitude and duration is generated each time that the input amplitude exceeds a threshold level: a dead time is arranged to prevent multiple registrations from a single echo complex. If the pulse duration is less than that corresponding to the resolution of the system, this processing scheme gives an apparently enhanced resolution, and it is particularly suited to certain organ mapping applications. This improvement, of course, is illusory. Recently, however, it has become apparent that much useful clinical data which otherwise would be lost, is obtained from B-scans in which echo amplitude information is retained in the form of a gray scale. This requires that the dynamic range of the image brightness should be sufficiently wide to convey some indication of the amplitudes of the echoes arising from within tissue structures, whilst simultaneously showing the stronger echoes from organ boundaries. The effect is further enhanced if the video amplifier has a logarithmic characteristic, and if the video signal has added to it a differentiated version of itself [5]. A typical scan is shown in Fig. 3.

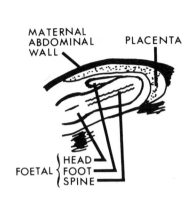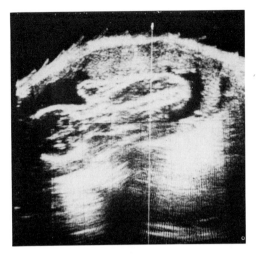

Fig. 3 Gray scale scan showing longitudinal section through a uterus with a 26 week foetus.

One result of this is to improve the resolution of the system in terms of its ability to separate the echoes from targets situated close together. This is because the registrations of the echoes are graded in brightness, being most intense at their centres. Consequently, the existence of two targets may be perceived as two brighter spots against an illuminated background, whilst they would appear coalesced on a display of smaller dynamic range.

There are two principal methods by which gray scale scans are obtained nowadays. The first uses a conventional cathode-ray tube with photographic recording. The dynamic range for brightness modulation of this type of tube is about 20 dB, and the analogue signal can be used to perform this function. Alternatively, a pulse of fixed amplitude may be generated, with a duration proportional to the amplitude of the echo; this is more satisfactory being both linear and capable of a wider dynamic range, provided that the maximum duration of the pulse is less than about one tenth of the deflection time corresponding to one spot diameter. The photographic conditions need careful adjustment. The brightness of the display is set so that the timebase line is just visible. For a given speed of film, the size of lens aperture determines the contrast of the image, so that a smaller stop (larger f-number) corresponds to a wider dynamic range. The system sensitivity is analogous to the illumination of the scene in conventional photography.

The second method of gray-scale scanning involves the use of a scan conversion memory tube. This consists of an evacuated tube containing a silicon — silicon oxide storage surface, and electron guns for writing and for reading. (In some designs, a single gun is used alternately for these two functions.) In the writing process, a charge pattern is deposited on the storage surface. Non-destructive reading is accomplished by the corresponding modulation of the scanning electron beam. The store may be erased by removing the charge pattern. The instrument was originally developed for converting television signals from one line standard to another. In two-dimensional ultrasonic B-scanning, the writing gun is controlled in the same way as that in the cathode-ray tube display of a conventional system. The stored image may be displayed continuously on a standard television monitor. The dynamic range is more than 50 dB, and so the required gray scale image can be obtained by adjustment of the brightness and contrast controls of the monitor. In this way, the effects on the image of changes in the displayed dynamic range can be observed without the need to rescan the patient. The resolution is better than 1 000 lines, which is about twice as good as an ordinary cathode ray tube, and four times as good as a direct-view storage tube. The storage surface retains the maximum written amplitude, and has little tendency to integrate in systems designed for ultrasonic use. The stored image can be viewed for about 10 min, and selected parts of the image may be enlarged for detailed examination. The video signal may easily be inverted, so that the black and the white parts of the image are interchanged: this can help in the perception of very weak echoes.

Before the development of gray-scale techniques, diagnosis on the basis of echo amplitude data could be made from several scans made in the same plane but at differing levels of system sensitivity. Thus, there is a tendency for cirrhotic liver to give rise to echoes of greater amplitude than those of normal liver [6]. What has been made easier by gray-scaling, however, is the recognition of small, isolated areas of abnormality, such as liver metastases [7]. An additional advantage of the scan conversion memory is that less skill is required in scanning, since the tendency to dwell momentarily at the end of each of the many arcing motions which combine to form a compound scan does not cause "coning" of the image.

DOPPLER SYSTEMS: SIGNAL ANALYSIS

The Doppler shift in the frequency of a backscattered ultrasonic wave of low megahertz frequency lies in the audible range at moderate reflector velocities. For example, a 2 MHz transmitted wave is shifted in frequency by about 260 Hz as a result of reflection from a surface moving at a velocity of 100 mm s^{-1} in a direction parallel to the ultrasonic beam. The shift in a frequency is upwards when the reflector is moving towards the transducer, and vice versa.

The most common application of ultrasonic Doppler techniques is in the detection of foetal heart pulsations [1]. In this procedure, familiar in almost every obstetric hospital, the probe - which contains transmitting and receiving transducers mounted side-by-side - is placed on the maternal abdomen, and the ultrasonic beam is directed towards the foetus. It is generally possible to hear the Doppler-shifted signals after about the twelfth week of pregnancy.

The Doppler method is also used in the study of blood flow. For peripheral vascular investigation, frequencies of 8-10 MHz are usual. Apart from merely listening to the Doppler-shifted signals from the moving blood, there are two distinct methods of analysis. The first depends on the zero-crossing frequency meter. There is no doubt that this system would be entirely satisfactory if all the blood flowed at an equal velocity along a uniform tube. In practice, however, the flow profile is likely to be parabolic, the flow may reverse during parts of the cardiac cycle, and the ultrasonic beam may pass through other vessels in addition to the one in which it is desired to study the flow. Therefore, results obtained with the zero-crossing detector must be interpreted with caution. The difficulties arise because the output of the detector can have only one value at any particular time, whilst the Doppler-shifted signals may extend over a spectrum of frequencies. Generally, it is the value of the maximum velocity at any instant which is of most interest. If the high-frequency components are of low amplitude, they "ride" on low-frequency components with the result that they do not all cross zero [8]. Consequently there is a tendency for the zero-crossing meter to read low. The difficulty may be minimised by the use of a filter which introduces an increasing loss with decreasing frequency. The statistical basis for this intuitively sensible treatment is discussed elsewhere [9].

The difficulties experienced with the zero-crossing detector can be almost entirely avoided by the use of the sound spectrograph for analysis [10]. The sound spectrograph is an instrument which generates a recording in which time and frequency are represented on the x and y axes respectively, and the corresponding energy densities are represented by the degree of blackening. A typical recording is shown in Fig. 4. The simultaneous occurrence of different flow velocities may be easily perceived, and the envelope of the spectrum corresponds to the

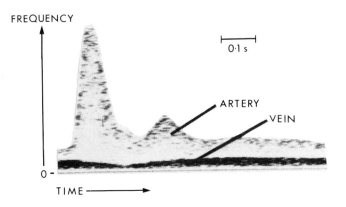

Fig. 4. Frequency spectrum showing separation of Doppler-shifted signals from an artery and a vein.

maximum flow velocity — which, in an ideal situation, is what would be indicated by a zero-crossing detector. Ordinary spectrographs use a bandpass filter which is swept through the range of frequencies under investigation, whilst a recording of the signals to be analysed is repeated by means of a tape loop. This type of instrument cannot operate in real time. Real-time spectrographs have been developed, however, either based on the use of a bank of bandpass filters each with its own read-out channel [11], or involving computer techniques.

REFERENCES

1 Wells, P.N.T. (1969). "Physical principles of ultrasonic diagnosis". Academic Press, London and New York.
2 Wells, P.N.T. (1971). "The standardisation of electronic systems in pulse-echo diagnosis". In "Ultrasonographia Medica", ed. J. Bock et al., Vol. II, pp. 29-37. Weiner Medizinischen Akademie, Vienna.
3 Wells, P.N.T. (1974). "The receiver in the pulse-echo system". In "Ultrasonics in Medicine", ed. M. de Vlieger et al., pp. 30-6. Excerpta Medica, Amsterdam; American Elsevier New York.
4 Kossoff, G. (1963). "Design of narrow-beamwidth transducers". J. acoust. Soc. Am., 35, 905-12.
5 Kossoff, G. (1972). "Improved techniques in cross sectional echography". Ultrasonics, 10, 221-7.
6 Wells P.N.T. (1971). "Physical factors controlling the diagnostic value of two-dimensional ultrasonic liver scans". In "Ultrasonographia Medica", ed. J. Bock et al., Vol.I, pp. 163-76. Weiner Medizinischen Akademie, Vienna.

7 Taylor, K.J.W., Carpenter, D.A., and McCready, V.R. (1973). "Gray scale echography in the diagnosis of intrahepatic disease". J. clin. Ultrasound, 1, 284-7.
8 Reneman, R.S. and Spencer, M.P. (1974). "Difficulties in processing of an analogue Doppler flow signal; with special reference to zero-crossing meters and quantification". In "Cardiovascular Applications of Ultrasound", ed. R.S. Reneman, pp. 32-42. North-Holland, Amsterdam; American Elsevier, New York.
9 Flax, S.W., Webster, J.G., and Updike, S.J. (1971). "Statistical evaluation of the Doppler ultrasonic blood flowmeter". Instr. Soc. Am. Trans., 10, 1-20.
10 Gosling, R.G., King, D.H., Newman, D.L., and Woodcock, J.P. (1969). "Transcutaneous measurement of arterial blood-velocity by ultrasound". In "Ultrasonics for Industry", pp. 16-23. IPC Business Press, Guildford.
11 Light, L.H. (1972). "Ultrasonic Doppler techniques in blood velocity measurement". In "Fluid Dynamic Measurements in the Industrial and Medical Environments", ed. D.J. Cockrell, Vol. 1, pp. 332-9. Leicester University Press, Leicester.

RADIONUCLIDE IMAGING - A QUICK SCAN THROUGH

J. A. McINTOSH

CHIEF PHYSICIST

Medical Physics Dept., Walsgrave Hospital, COVENTRY

Radionuclides have been used diagnostically as a clinical aid for more than thirty years but their usefulness has greatly increased since instruments such as rectilinear scanners and Anger Gamma Cameras were first developed less than twenty years ago. The technique of radio nuclide scanning consists of drawing out the distribution of radioactivity within the body after the administration of a radiopharmaceutical.

The rectilinear scanner was the first imaging device to make a real impact. The detector head, consisting of a sodium iodide crystal, photomultiplier and collimator moves relative to a couch at a uniform speed so that all areas are sampled for the same period and the entire organ is covered progressively line by line.

The present generation of scanners may have one, two or three heads and some are capable of such sophistication as transverse tomograms. However, no matter how many heads or what views are required to be taken, the information from the head is always fed to associated electronic equipment where it is processed to a greater or less extent and the results displayed. It is difficult to give a figure for resolution as the final resolution obtained depends so much on the techniques employed at the various centres. In practice about 0.5cms. is generally possible, however, abnormalities smaller than 1cm. diameter will not be resolved.

The other important imaging instrument is the Anger Gamma Camera. This consists essentially of a large sodium iodide crystal up to 33cms. in diameter and 1cm. thick, with as many as 37 photomultipliers. Between crystal and photomultiplier tubes there is an optical light guide. There is a multi-channel collimator consisting of hundreds of parallel holes separated by lead between the patient and the crystal. Gamma rays coming from the patient, which travel up the vertical channel of the collimator, will cause scintillation on the sodium iodide crystal. Those not travelling vertical will be absorbed by the lead septa. The photomultiplier tubes detect the scintillation and each tube produces a signal proportional to the intensity of the light and its location. The output of the photomultipliers are electronically analogued to give positional information.

The resultant output is fed to a storage oscilloscope where the positional information is fed to the X and Y plates and an event is seen on a screen at a point which corresponds to the position of the original event in the crystal. A Polaroid camera set at live exposure can photograph the events over a fixed time. Again, as with scanners, more sophisticated storage and memory units may be used in conjunction with a small computer so that further analysis and processing can take place.

Scanning was handicapped for a considerable time because of the lack of a radionuclide of suitable half-life and energy. Fortunately, the Gods were on the side of the physicists when Technetium was produced. This nuclide has a suitably short half-life but above all emits gamma quanta of 140 KeV. Sodium iodide also has its maximum detection efficiency around 140 KeV, this therefore resulted in massive strides forward in radionuclide imaging. Fortunate indeed, that Technetium also can be easily tagged to many pharmaceuticals again resulting in rapid development of radiopharmaceuticals suitable for imaging many organs.

It is in the development of better and more specific radiopharmaceuticals that the most outstanding advances will be made in the near future. Instrumentation has rapidly improved over the last two or three years but there has been a lack of development of really first class specific radiopharmaceuticals. For example, if a radiopharmaceutical could be developed to image the pancreas as well as diphosphonate does the bone, gastro-enterologists would be delighted. With a better understanding of the reasons for a particular distribution of a radiopharmaceutical within an organ and with more specific radiopharmaceuticals, the technique of radionuclide imaging will lead to more specific diagnosis and better differential diagnosis; both these requirements are essential to make radionuclide scanning a really viable diagnostic technique in the future.

The method of display of radionuclide scan data is of the utmost importance if assessment is to be made by a human observer and the final display must give the maximum assistance to the observer if the interpretation is to be rapid and accurate.

Many techniques have been used in practice for scanners. There have been (i) black marks on white paper, (ii) coloured marks on white paper, (iii) monochrome photographic recording, (iv) coloured photographic recording, (v) digital displays, both colour and black and white. For Gamma Cameras we have had (a) picture usually stored on a photograph, from a cathode ray tube, or (b) digital displays, black and white or colour.

It is extremely difficult to lay down a hard and fast rule as to which display ought to be used as the method of interpretation is so subjective, and many observers will stick to the display they have become used to. Because of the greater dynamic range possible in colour it is obvious that whichever intermediate process is carried out the final display is best presented in colour form. The requirement is therefore for a quantitative multi-level display system to enable a visual assessment of the data from scanners or cameras to be made, either in its raw form or in its computer processed form.

It is generally accepted that the need for processing is very much dependent upon the diagnostic technique being performed but in most investigations a limited degree of smoothing is required. This however, can generally be simply done in a simple hard wired system built into the scanner or the colour print out. For a straight forward rectilinear scan of the brain expensive computers and processors are a luxury and of doubtful clinical value: however, when more sophisticated scanning techniques are required such as transverse section scanning, some form of off-line computer is essential.

For many years the Anger Gamma Camera was an inferior instrument to the scanner because of three main reasons: (a) poor resolution, (b) poor uniformity, and (c) poor display.

The resolution and uniformity of present cameras shows great improvement compared with the past and one can no longer say that a scanner has a superior resolution to a camera. However, the one big handicap of the camera is that without some form of processor or even a small dedicated computer, the field uniformity and the final display lack the quality essential for good diagnosis. Both problems can be solved with small inexpensive hard wired processors and provided that only static work is required, in fact provided only work similar to that done on a scanner is to be undertaken, there is absolutely no need for large expensive processors or computers. The fact that a single view can be taken much quicker on a camera that on a scanner is extremely useful on many occasions as it is often desirable to scan immediately after injection to assist in the differential diagnosis of, for example, a brain lesion. This is easily done on a camera and several views can be taken at short intervals of time, without highly sophisticated computer processing.

On the other hand, if dynamic investigations are to be performed one is not off first base without a fairly sophisticated computer back-up to the camera. Dynamic investigations are becoming increasingly more popular in differential diagnosis of brain lesions, renograms, cardiac, lung and liver studies. The rate at which the radiopharmaceutical is picked up, or filtered out, or the rate of blood flow, are all factors which can be readily calculated using a Gamma Camera computer and processing unit. At present, however, although these investigations have proved extremely useful clinically, the £70,000 required for such a set up is not justified except in the large centres.

Should radionuclide imaging be a technique available to all district general hospitals? Personally I don't think so. Even the simple rectilinear scanner or a Gamma Camera costing between £15,000 and £20,000 are expensive pieces of equipment and their running costs are relatively high. Larger centres ought to be chosen and they should provide a service on a sub-regional basis. In this way one makes the optimum use of equipment and staff and prevents standards falling which they are apt to do in areas where experienced physicists, clinicians and technicians are not always present.

There is also considerable controversy in the value and suitability of many of the more highly sophisticated processors and displays. Many physicists feel that some manufacturers have developed beautiful display systems without enough consideration of perception theory. Physicists and psychologists must collaborate and understand fully the problems associated with visual perception and having done this design a display properly suited to the human eye.

It is imperative that many of the larger centres have large soft-wire computers linked to their detection systems in order to develop new programmes and techniques but it may be that in the medium sized and smaller centres where physicists are harassed and overworked, that small hard-wired systems would be more suitable. There are such systems, of course, available commercially at this time, but care must be taken so that the most useful one is purchased. There are several totally unsuited for the work of a busy imaging department.

As already mentioned, it is in the field of radiopharmaceuticals that advances are most likely to occur. Certain organs such as the pancreas, are waiting to be imaged but as yet the pharmaceutical has not been found. Gallium and indium labelled bleomycin are two tumour seeking pharmaceuticals of more recent origin but they are far from ideal. One must try to produce radiopharmaceuticals which are more specific in their destination and also radiopharmaceuticals to aid differential diagnosis. Associated with this is the problem of understanding the physiological path taken by the radiopharmaceutical and when this is more clearly understood more detailed diagnostic information will be available.

The improvements which have been made recently in colour displays will I am sure continue, and such techniques as early dynamic studies in investigations of all organs and transverse tomograms will considerably assist the diagnostician in making accurate assessments of the region studied.

Detectors using materials other than sodium iodide are being tried, but at present these solid state detectors have not proved very successful, because although their resolution is excellent their sensitivity and convenience is relatively poor. It may be that multi-wired proportioned counters are less restricted to technological development and this should make them more commercially viable for certain sophisticated applications.

Pattern recognition by computers would remove the subjective assessment of the diagnostician but as yet this technique is not applied routinely although many centres are working on it. Undoubtedly, there is scope here and soon the final assessment by the observer will be backed up by a computer prediction.

This is fine but it must be remembered at all times that the end product must facilitate an accurate assessment of the radionuclide image leading to a differential diagnosis of the region mapped out and all paths must be directed towards this goal.

THERMOGRAPHY IN THE INVESTIGATION OF BREAST CANCER

A.L. Evans, W.B. James and M. Davison

Department of Radiology, Southern General Hospital, Glasgow, and Department of Clinical Physics and Bio-Engineering, West of Scotland Health Boards, Glasgow

The fundamental concept used in thermography is that skin temperature abnormalities are manifestations of underlying pathology. This has been known since the earliest days of medicine – Hippocrates was aware of the high left-right symmetry of skin temperature in the human body. Until recently, skin temperature had to be estimated by touch – this is still a good method; in good circumstances the hand can detect $1^{\circ}C$ differences in skin temperature. Accurate spot temperature readings can now be made with thermocouples, thermistors or with radiometers. The next step – the presentation of an image of skin temperature distribution – was greatly assisted by funds injected into the military aspects of temperature displays.

The intensity of infra-red radiation emitted by the skin is a measure of the skin temperature. The thermographic camera forms an image of the emission of infra-red radiation from the skin (Figure 1). The radiation of wavelength up to 5.5 μm is detected by indium antimonide cooled to liquid nitrogen temperatures. The electrical signal from the detector is amplified before it is used to modulate the intensity of the spot on a cathode ray tube. By making the radiation from different parts of an object fall upon the detector and by corresponding movement of the oscilloscope spot an image is formed of the surface temperature of the object.

A permanent record may be made of the image in several ways. The simplest way is to take a black and white polaroid or 35 mm photograph of the oscilloscope screen. Most systems can display isothermal lines on the image, and, by interposing colour filters, a temperature contour map can be created. Several groups – especially in the United Kingdom – are engaged in digitising the thermograms and in the computer processing of the displays. Provided one has the money to spend, considerable sophistication can be attained in the

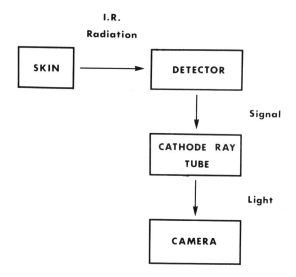

Figure 1. Block diagram of a thermographic camera.

acquisition and display of skin temperature images. Does the information obtained justify the expense and effort?

Thermography is most commonly used in the investigation of breast disease. Normal breast thermograms have been well documented by several workers notably Draper and Jones (1969) and Bourjat and Gautherie (1972). The patterns are essentially of two types - the avascular breast which appears uniformly cool and the vascular breast in which the superficial veins contribute to a distinct temperature pattern (Figure 2a). Important points to note are that the breasts are quite symmetrical and the fact that each woman's pattern remains constant over her lifetime (Stark and Way, 1974; Phillips and Lloyd Williams, 1974).

In 1956 Lawson observed that the skin over malignant tumours of the breast is warmer than on the opposite side (Figure 2b). Since that time, several criteria for malignancy have become established (Amalric, 1974): hypervascularisation, hot spot of greater than $3^{\circ}C$, hyperthermia of the whole breast greater than $2^{\circ}C$, the edge sign. Unfortunately the basis for these criteria is experience rather than scientific method.

In Glasgow we have made an approach to the objective evaluation of thermograms (Feasey, Evans and James, 1975). We have measured differences in temperature between the affected breast and the normal breast using the following factors : hot spot temperature, pattern temperature, and nipple temperature. We have also assessed the prominence of the pattern and the background temperature; for our survey

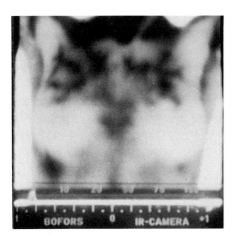 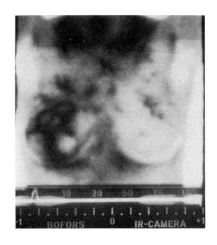

Figure 2. a) Left; the thermographic appearance of normal breasts.
b) Right; the skin is warmer over a malignant tumour in the right
breast. The black areas are the hot areas in this presentation.

the last two factors were assessed subjectively, but we are now in
a position to measure these factors quantitatively.

Our survey was made on 249 thermograms; 58 normal women, 102
benign and 89 malignant lesions, all of which were proven histolog-
ically. By taking batches containing equal numbers of normals,
benigns and carcinomas the thermograms were read completely blind
with an equal chance of any particular one being normal, benign or
malignant. Each thermogram was subsequently assigned a score according to the temperature differences recorded. Figure 3 shows histograms of the three groups - normal, benign and malignant - at different thermographic score values. It is clear that thermography can
not be used to differentiate benign and malignant lesions. Its use
in routine diagnostic departments is therefore to be discouraged.

Our survey also gives information about the effectiveness of
thermography in picking out malignant cases from a well woman population - that is, mass screening for breast cancer. Figure 3 shows
that the false negative rate is 31 per cent - carcinomas with negative thermograms - and the false positive rate is 33 per cent -
normals with positive thermograms. These rates are higher than most
of those quoted in the literature (see for example Amalric, 1974
and Jones, 1973); it must be stressed that this work is an attempt
to measure the effectiveness of thermography under strictly defined
conditions of observer bias.

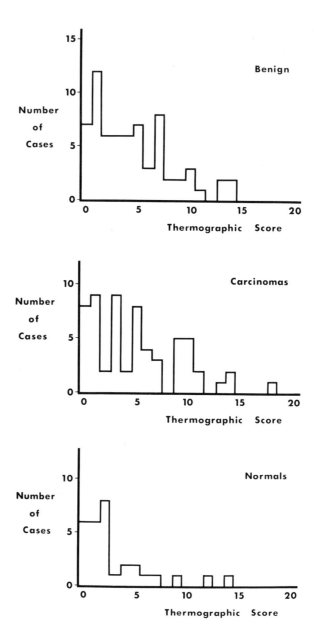

Figure 3. Histograms of the number of cases at each thermographic score value for the normal, benign and malignant groups.

If we used thermography as an initial screening technique with these false positive and false negative rates, a 2 carcinomas in 1000 well woman population could be concentrated to a 4.7 in 1000 high risk group for further study i.e. clinical examination and mammography. This procedure would reduce the number of people to be further examined by a factor of three. An incidence of 0.9 per 1000 would remain in the population "passed" by the initial screening.

A scheme for the screening clinic is shown in Figure 4. The receptionist records the patient's name on arrival at the clinic. The patient undresses to the waist and cools for 15 minutes before entering the thermography room. She is accurately positioned by a radiographer who "takes the picture" - that is, sends the image data into the computer. The woman dresses, returns to the reception area where she is given the result. This is in one of three forms : 1. Cleared. 2. Come back in 3 months. 3. An appointment for a clinical examination and mammography. These correspond to a negative, equivocal and a positive thermography interpretation.

The scheme is certainly possible but is it worth it? One unit examining 10 women per hour could manage 10,000 per year. A city the size of Glasgow would need 20 units to screen every woman every year. The thermography alone would therefore cost somewhere in the region of £300,000 per year. This would select a third of the screened population for further examination by a clinician and for mammography. This latter service would cost over £800,000 per annum. So the total cost would be £1.1 m per annum. The result would be the finding of 300 carcinomas perhaps one year earlier than they would have presented anyway.

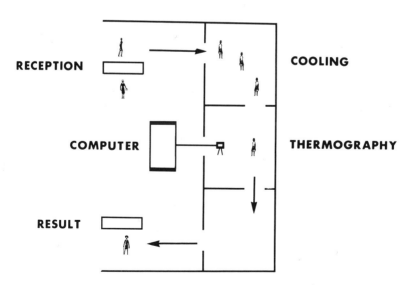

Figure 4. A screening clinic using thermography.

We are not aware of any statistically valid evidence that present treatments modify the natural history of breast cancer. Even so, a screening programme might still be justified on economic grounds if much simpler therapy was adopted in "early" carcinoma - "lumpectomy" for example. The cost of a screening programme would have to be balanced against possible saving in the cost of therapy.

In summary, if thermography is used in a manner similar to that described, we can conclude that :
1. Thermography has no place as a diagnostic technique in breast cancer.
2. A screening programme to produce a high risk population for breast disease is certainly feasible albeit very expensive. We do not consider such a programme appropriate for breast cancer.
3. Further studies are required to improve the sensitivity and specificity of thermography and to examine its usefulness as a prognostic instrument.

References

Amalric, R., Spitalier, J.M., Giraud, D., Altschuler, C. (1974). Telethermography in diagnosis of breast diseases. In Proceedings of the 1st European Congress on Thermography. Karger, Basel.

Bourjat, P. and Gautherie, M. (1972). Thermography of mammary carcinomas. Electromedica, $\underline{1}$, 17.

Draper, J.W. and Jones, C.H. (1969). Thermal patterns of the female breast. Br. J. Radiol. $\underline{42}$, 401.

Feasey, C.F., Evans, A.L. and James, W.B. (1975). Thermography in breast carcinoma : results of a blind reading trial. Br. J. Radiol. (In press).

Jones, C.H. (1973). Detection of breast lesions : Thermography. In Modern Trends in Oncology, ed. R.W. Raven. Butterworths, London.

Lawson, R.N. (1956). Implications of surface temperatures in the diagnosis of breast cancers. Can. Med. Assoc. J., $\underline{75}$, 309.

Phillips, B.H. and Lloyd Williams, K. (1974). The clinical use of thermography. British Journal of Hospital Medicine, November Equipment Supplement.

Stark, A.M. and Way, S. (1974). The use of Thermovision in the detection of early breast cancer. Cancer, $\underline{33}$, 1664.

PERSPECTIVES IN RADIODIAGNOSIS

LOUIS KREEL

CONSULTANT RADIOLOGIST, NORTHWICK PARK HOSPITAL
& HEAD OF RADIOLOGY, CLINICAL RESEARCH CENTRE
WATFORD ROAD, HARROW, MIDDLESEX, U.K.

It has been estimated that the number of radiological investigations increases at about the rate of 10% annually, (Ashley et al, 1972). This is only for conventional radiological examinations and does not include the introduction of newer methods, such as isotope scanning or ultrasonography. The increasing cost of radiology departments is due not only to these factors or, for that matter, to the obvious increasing cost of film and chemicals or rising salaries. There is for instance an overall rise in expectations and standards on the part of the medical profession and patients, which is a natural feature of industrialised societies. We are all striving for perfection and seldom give a thought to the effects this has on public expenditure. While individual departments and radiologists do not directly control and feel responsible for their own budgets, this will continue to be so.

The cost of these examinations is not the only consideration, but there is also the unresolved issue of the radiation hazard from diagnostic procedures. The possibility of induction of malignancy and genetic abnormalities have been commented upon repeatedly (ICRP report, 1970). This is no longer just a question of the effects on radiation workers but also on individual patients and whole population groups (Kitabatake et al, 1973). A first step in the right direction in this regard is the effective implementation of the 10 day rule (Warrick, 1973) and every precaution must be taken to prevent irradiation during pregnancy, particularly in the earliest stages. The implications of these arguments are obvious. The investigation of a patient to obtain an accurate diagnosis must be a step-wise process and not a blunderbuss affair. These must proceed from the simple, least expensive and least traumatic to the complex and hazardous procedures and must not be divorced from the clinical management of the patient.

Disease of the biliary tract can be taken to illustrate this point. There are many clinical and biochemical pointers to pathology of the biliary system. Basically, and perhaps looking at this problem in too simplistic a way, what is required is to know whether the patient has evidence of gall stones, obstruction to the duct system, chronic cholecystitis, adenomyomatosis or, if one believes in the entity, dyskinesia of the gall bladder. Gall stones may be shown on a plain film of the abdomen as a chance finding when a film is taken for some other reason, such as the control film for a pyelogram or barium enema. Unsuspected gall stones have in fact, been found in 10-15% of women over the age of 50 years. The management of these individuals presents a problem as nearly half will develop gall bladder disease within ten years (Wenckert & Robertson, 1966).

From the point of view of screening procedures, should a routine abdominal film be offered to all women over 50 years of age and, when discovered, should they then be offered surgery ? At present, however, most patients with biliary tract disease present with a suggestive clinical picture. In these cases, the discovery of unequivocal evidence of gall stones is sufficient evidence for recommending elective surgery. Of course, by unequivocal evidence, one means single or multiple, ring or laminated opacities maintaining a constant and close relationship to the liver margin. If these opacities are also faceted, this is even stronger evidence that they are gall stones. Only if the opacities are not as typical as this or none are shown on the plain film should an oral cholecystogram be done. It is now well-established that 2 G (4 tablets) of iopanoic acid is effective and side effects minimal at this dose, but if the gall bladder does not show after 14 hours, this dose should be repeated and a further film taken the following day. If the gall bladder is still not shown, a dose of calcium ipodate must then be given and a film taken 2 - 4 hours later. If this regime is carried out, and in the absence of vomiting, diarrhoea, liver disease or cholecystectomy, non-visualisation of the gall bladder indicates a diseased organ to an accuracy of 95% (Hodgson & Baker, 1959), which is, by all standards a good biological and clinical test.

The procedure can be streamlined in that all cases requiring an oral cholecystogram can, at the outset, be given the two doses, each to be taken on successive evenings, with the saving of a significant number of double visits and double examinations. Furthermore, in those cases that have non-visualisation, the accuracy can be further increased by a repeat examination. As in most centres the operative waiting time is months rather than weeks, a final check cholecystogram can be done and in these circumstances the accuracy rate becomes 99%.

What then should the logical approach to intravenous cholangiography be in the non-visualised gall bladder after oral cholecystography ? The contrast agents used for this intravenous procedure have the most untoward side-effects of all those presently used, and furthermore it is now widely recognised that operative cholangiography is an essential adjunct to biliary surgery. It must also be recognised that, even in the best hands, something like 50% of stones will not be seen on the intravenous cholangiogram.

The toxicity of the contrast agent, the relative inaccuracy of the examination and the routine use of operative cholangiography can only mean that, in the vast majority of cases, non-visualisation of the gall bladder on oral cholecystography is no longer an indication for an intravenous cholangiogram. This does not mean there is no place for intravenous cholangiography which is still the method of choice in patients who have had cholecystectomies, and in whom there is a recurrence of symptoms indicating disease of the biliary tract.

The patient presenting with "obstructive" jaundice falls into quite a different diagnostic situation. Oral cholecystography or intravenous cholangiography are unlikely to produce helpful information and a laparotomy in those cases shown to have "medical" jaundice can be hazardous. It therefore becomes essential to separate cases of non-obstructive (medical) jaundice from obstructive (surgical) cases. To be effective in terms of patient management the major ducts must be demonstrated. They will then be shown to be either of normal calibre or dilated. If the bile ducts are dilated then the level of obstruction must be demonstrated, (Kreel, 1973).

In this context the least complicated examinations are also the least accurate, but because they are simple, must be done first. The chest radiograph and plain film of the abdomen must of course be available, but are rarely discriminating. However, the barium meal done in such a way as to produce a double contrast duodenogram can demonstrate the impression of a dilated common bile duct or a pancreatic carcinoma and will also exclude an intrinsic lesion of the stomach or duodenum. If ultrasound is available it could be used as confirmatory evidence of the presence of dilated bile ducts. Should these examinations show that the duct system is dilated, laparotomy will follow but should be preceded by percutaneous cholangiography to show the site of the obstruction, its pathology and possibly whether 'intrahepatic lesions are also present. A markedly enlarged liver or ascites will, of course, require to be taken into account and the plan of diagnostic management varied accordingly.

However, if the above-mentioned investigations are negative there may still be a dilated duct system but it then also becomes essential to show whether there is in fact a normal duct system. The endoscopic retrograde cholangio-pancreaticogram (E.R.C.P.) is particularly valuable in this respect. It is, however, expensive in terms of instrumentation and manpower and the expertise is as yet not available in all general hospitals.

The percutaneous transhepatic cholangiogram done with a fine needle-catheter system, and exploring the duct system with injections of contrast medium rather than aspiration of bile will succeed in most cases (Okuda et al, 1974). This method is more widely available and if a normal duct system is found it will save the patient an unnecessary and possibly hazardous operation. In the vast majority of cases, the duct system needs to be shown by only one method but this must be by an effective method and then the other radiological information becomes irrelevant. This means that oral cholecystography, intravenous cholangiography, operative cholangiography and arteriography will then not need to be done in most cases of 'obstructive' jaundice.

Similar arguments based on management-orientated lines of investigation have shown that the pyelogram in hypertension, the barium meal in the acute phase of haematemasis and the barium follow-through examination in malabsorption must not be used as a screening procedure but for the identification of specific abnormalities after other investigations, particularly biochemical, have been performed. In this way considerably fewer investigations will be done without loss of clinical information.

It is also to be remembered that in geriatric patients who are too frail or have cardio-respiratory disease which excludes major surgery, it is pointless undertaking investigations which will lead to diagnoses requiring major surgery. As has been said previously, these radiological procedures are expensive, unpleasant to the patient and time-consuming. If they add nothing to the clinical management then they are unjustified and only add to already overstretched waiting lists.

Our attention must be directed not only to the contrast studies but also to the more simple examinations such as chest radiography. Routine annual chest radiographs are still demanded by many institutions, schools, hospitals and industrial employers. It has also become current practice to have a routine chest radiograph as a pre-operative procedure irrespective of the age of the patient or whether it is for a minor or major operation. With the elimination of tuberculosis as a major hazard, apart from specific groups such as recent immigrants, diabetics and the elderly, the main reason for chest radiography as a screening procedure has been eliminated. Certainly in adolescents or young adults the pick-up rate is virtually negligible (Sagel et al, 1974) and furthermore, a tuberculin test is a cheaper and far more effective method (Jacobs, 1974).

It has also been shown that the chest radiograph as a routine screening procedure, even when taken at six monthly intervals, does not substantially alter the prognosis in bronchial carcinoma (Boucot & Weiss, 1973). In the under 40-year olds, the lateral radiograph, again as a screening procedure in the asymptomatic patients, makes a negligible contribution to the detection of disease (Sagel et al, 1974). The evidence now overwhelmingly indicates that chest radiography as a routine screening procedure in the adolescent and young adult and the routine use of the lateral film in the under 40-year old is no longer justified in developed countries. While the elimination of unnecessary exposure to radiation must continue to be a major function of radiologists, it is equally important to obtain maximum information from each examination, particularly by being aware of recent advances. The double contrast barium meal can be taken as an example. It is now possible, by using the Japanese technique (Shirakabe et al, 1971 : Kreel et al, 1974) to detect tiny ulcers, erosive gastritis and surface tumours as small as 1 - 2 cm. By using this method together with newer film/screen combinations, although more films are taken, radiation per examination can be halved. However, to be sure that these newer techniques are reliable requires not only a meticulous attention to detail but also a thorough appreciation of the details of the radiological signs shown. To do this, the radiologist must work closely not only with the

clinicians but also with the histo-pathologist. It is
essential that the endoscopist, radiologist and histo-
pathologist learn to speak the same language and learn
to appreciate each others problems and limitations as
well as their own.

While the problems of cost-effectiveness and medical audit
are receiving considerable attention, while refinements
of older methods give new information and while newer
techniques are being introduced, there is also the ever-
present possibility of new and revolutionary equipment
being introduced. Two such advances have occurred in
radiodiagnosis in the last few years. These are of course
the 'grey-scale' in ultrasonics and the EMI scanner using
X-rays. The introduction of the grey-scale to ultrasonics
has made it possible to obtain pictures which are more
and more like conventional anatomical displays. This is,
of course, best illustrated with the study of the foetus
in which the ventricles of the brain, the spinal cord,
the heart and mitral valve, and the umbilical cord can
now be shown as definite, recognisable anatomical
structures. The next few years will almost certainly see
an explosion of diagnostic information from this
instrument.

The EMI scanner or transverse axial tomography using
computerisation of the recorded data greatly increases
the yield of information from the Roentgen-tube. It is
now possible to ascribe relative tissue densities, not
just to fat, muscle and bone but also to blood, serous
fluids and tumours. These tissue densities can be further
enhanced by the use of intravenous contrast agents and
probably also intestinal contrast substances. At present,
experience is based on intracerebral lesions. A 'body
machine' will be available soon. It is, of course,
impossible to predict its place in the scheme of
anatomical diagnostic procedure but it is surely not too
much to hope that it will make a very real contribution.

There can be little doubt, therefore, that the prospects
in diagnostic radiology are exciting. However, this
excitement must not be allowed to obscure or hide many
of the real problems which face medicine and radiologists
in particular. Too much work of greater and greater
complexity chases too few trained personnel, who in any
case are only too liable to develop "tunnel vision". The
rational use of diagnostic resources has been mentioned,
as has the increased yield from conventional methods,
as well as the equipment of the future, but as yet, little
has been said about the 'soft-ware'.

The problems of the Health Service, the effects of a 38 or 40 hour week and the state of the economy will certainly affect us all. While recognising that it is impossible to divorce this from our daily professional activities there are two, much more parochial questions which must be answered. Can the role of the radiographers remain unaltered ? Must the radiologist continue to report every examination passing through the department, including all films from the Accident and Emergency departments ? Briefly, in considering the first question, it must be recognised that, in future, radiographers will be required to operate isotope scanning equipment, ultrasound and EMI scanners. It will inevitably mean even greater specialisation and, of course, yet more personnel. They may well then be required to give injections, particularly of isotopes and intravenous contrast agents and this would of course require the appropriate medico-legal recognition. If this kind of development occurs in radiology, how will this affect other workers in the sciences allied to medicine, including the nursing staff ?

It can just be mentioned in passing as a possible future trend that, in some centres in Japan, technicians perform barium meal examinations by taking a standard series of films during a standardised procedure. To turn to the work of radiologists, for one moment we can look at a problem at the other extreme. If the skills and expertise required of them has increased to such a degree (so the argument goes), then surely a large burden of routine must be lifted from them and what better than the routine of accident and emergency reporting ?

This viewpoint is to be deplored and would, to my mind, make for unsatisfactory hospital practice. Most accident and emergency departments are staffed by juniors, working under pressure but requiring a wide range of expertise. The only way to cope with this situation is to see that the back-up services are of high calibre and freely available. Not only must all films be reported, but I would suggest that the radiology of Accident and Emergency departments be served by consultants, rather than by junior specialist staff. This would go a long way to giving this very important aspect of hospital work adequate cover in both the medical and medico-legal sense.

The advances and problems in radiology reflect those in hospital practice and medicine as a whole. I personally feel optimistic as to the future of my own specialty within the National Health Service and its ability to provide the necessary expertise and good sense for the public at large.

REFERENCES

1. Ashley, J.S.A., Pasker, P. and Beresford, J.C. (1972)
   Lancet 1: 890

2. Boucot, K.R. and Weiss, W. (1973)
   Is curable lung cancer detected by semi-annual screening?
   Journal of the American Medical Association 224:1361

3. Hodgson, J.R. and Baker, H.L.Jnr. (1959)
   Newer concepts in cholecystography and cholangiography
   Postgraduate Medicine 26:283

4. Committee 3 of the ICRP (1970) - A report
   Protection against ionizing radiation from external sources
   ICRP Publication 15, New York, Pergamon Press

5. Jacobs, J.C. (1974)
   Chest X-ray screening for tuberculosis
   Journal of the American Medical Association 228:24

6. Kitabatake, T., Yokoyama, M., Sakka, M. & Koga, S. (1973)
   Estimation of benefit and radiation risk from mass chest radiography
   Radiology 109:37

7. Kreel, L. (1973)
   Radiology of the biliary system
   Clinics in Gastroenterology 2:185

8. Kreel, L., Herlinger, H. & Glanville, J. (1973)
   Technique of the double contrast barium meal with examples of correlation with endoscopy
   Clinical Radiology 24:307

9. Okuda, K., Kyuichi, T., Takeshi, E., Shintaro, K., Shigenobu, J., Kazuki, U., Toshiro, S., Yoshiro, K., Yoshio, F., Hirotaka, M., Hiromichi, M., Yutaka, S., Fusakuni, Y., Yasuhiko, M. (1974)
   Non-surgical, percutaneous transhepatic cholangiography diagnostic significance in medical problems of the liver
   Digestive Diseases 19 : No.1:36

10. Shirakabe, H. (1971)
    Double Contrast Studies of the Stomach
    Bunkodo Co. Ltd. Tokyo, Japan

11. Warrick, C.K. (1973)
    Radiology Now : The "10-day" rule
    British Journal of Radiology 46:933

12. Wenckert, A. & Robertson, B. (1966)
    Gastroenterology 50:376

PART III

New Diagnostic Techniques in Special Departments

MONITORING THE EEG IN LIVER DISEASE

B. MacGillivray, D. Wadbrook, P. M. Quilter

Royal Free Hospital

London

The liver is the main and essential organ for the conversion of foodstuffs into forms suitable for use by the body. It functions also as the main organ for the detoxication of noxious by-products of metabolism, drugs and other poisonous substances absorbed from the bowel. Severe malfunction of the liver results in the accumulation of toxic substances in the blood which in turn have a profound effect on the brain leading to coma and eventual death. This sequence of events has largely common clinical features irrespective of the precise cause of the liver disease.

Liver failure may occur acutely as in viral hepatitis or toxic necrosis (some industrial poisons, suicidal drug overdose) or more chronically as a sequel to previous infections, chronic malnutrition, alcoholism, and a variety of other conditions. Since the recuperative powers of the liver are considerable it is, in clinical practice, nearly always worthwhile instituting supportive measures, often of quite heroic proportions, to tide the body over the acute phases of the liver failure until some recovery of liver function takes place. This applies also in patients with chronic liver disease (cirrhosis or hardening of the liver) who may be temporarily precipitated into acute liver decompensation by some intercurrent infection, haemorrhage into the bowel, or a number of other transient phenomena. Such patients will die if untreated but can recover and live for several years if carefully managed.

Once a patient goes into coma, it becomes increasingly difficult to determine from the clinical features whether there is continued deterioration or some improvement in response to treatment. The biochemical correlates of liver failure are extremely complex

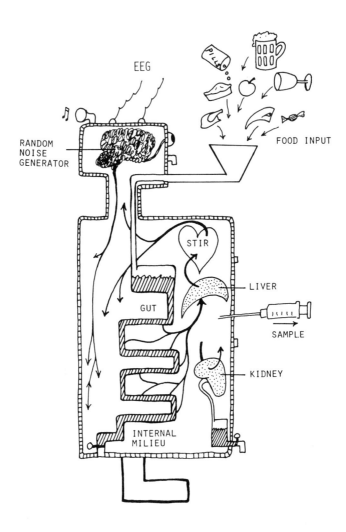

Fig.1 Schematic man to illustrate the central position of the liver in maintaining the stability of the internal milieu in the face of a random conglomeration of food inputs. Particular problems when the liver is diseased are caused by alcohol, protein, and drugs of various kinds. When the chemical environment of the brain (random noise generator) is disturbed, the EEG changes.

as might be expected from failure in an organ which is so central to the stability of the internal metabolic state. No single biochemical or toxic factor correlates with the patient's condition and indeed it is very likely that we are observing a multifactor phenomenon. One common feature is the function of the brain, which becomes increasingly impaired as the patient deteriorates. It is here that the EEG plays a useful role. The mechanisms of liver coma have been recently reviewed (Lunzer 1975) and also the nature of the EEG changes (MacGillivray, 1975).

Normal brain wave patterns (EEG) depend on a normal and stable chemical composition in the blood and tissue fluids from which the brain gains its nourishment. This 'internal milieu' is kept constant by a host of homeostatic mechanisms amongst which the functions of the liver and kidneys are essential (Fig. 1). Perturbations of this fluid environment (metabolic and toxic disease) alter the 'cerebral noise' or EEG. Usually these changes are non-specific. That is, the wave patterns are not specific to the particular disease, but they nonetheless often show clear 'dose/response' relations common to a particular disease or toxic state across different subjects. 'Dose' here refers to the factors, directly if known, or inferred from other observations, such as other chemical changes, or from clinical observations, for example the level of consciousness. 'Response' refers to some detectable change in the EEG.

In the case of liver failure where the 'dose' factors are as yet imprecisely defined and probably multiple, the best measure we have of 'dose' is the clinical state - a set of observations primarily dependent on the level of consciousness and the presence or absence of certain reflexes, but taking into account other factors such as the blood pressure, rate of respiration, temperature and so on. Despite the essentially qualitative nature of the observations, the experienced observer produces consistant estimations of practical value which also turn out to correlate remarkably well with an independent measure derived from the EEG (Fig. 2) as will be described. Having once established the general nature of these correlations, the EEG can be the more useful and reliable measure. Hence the value of monitoring the EEG in liver failure problems.

The essence of monitoring is to detect changes in state. To be useful, and more particularly acceptable in practice, the arrangements must be reasonably simple to implement, reliable and above all produce an output easily comprehended and instantly related to the clinical state. Whilst the raw EEG fulfils these demands to some extent (Fig. 2) interpretation requires some skill and considerable experience. Further, there are obvious advantages in having some quantifiable parameter. It should perhaps be remarked that where one is dealing with some systemic disorder of cerebral

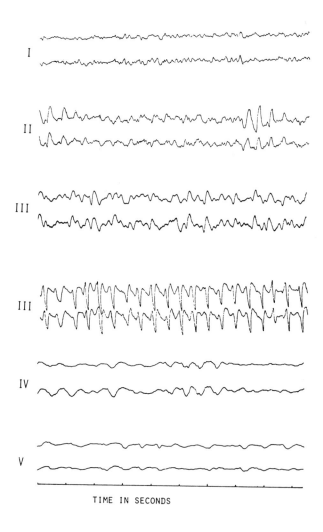

Fig. 2 Typical examples of EEG patterns recorded from patients in clinical coma grades I-V. The common feature is a gradual slowing of the dominant frequencies. There are two patterns of coma grade III, the lower 'triphasic wave' pattern occurs in about 30-50% of patients for reasons not known (possibly genetic). The two channels of EEG are recorded from wide spaced (12 cms) electrodes from the right central and parietal regions.

MONITORING THE EEG IN LIVER DISEASE

function it is usually feasible to obtain a good measure of the disturbances from a single EEG channel, provided one sticks to the same area of brain for all recordings. Advantages can also be taken of the differential input to the amplifiers so that each of the two recording electrodes can contribute to the output from two parts of the brain simultaneously.

In the past (MacGillivray, 1968, Kennedy et al 1973) we have used a set of broad band analogue filters to describe an amplitude frequency spectrum of the EEG signal displayed in the form of a five bar histogram for 10, 15 or 20 seconds periods or as a running average displayed on an oscilloscope or written out on a chart. The display was subsequently simplified further by computing the centre of gravity, first moment or mean frequency, of the spectrum as one component and the mean amplitude of the signal as a second component. As will be seen, neither of these components alone is quite sufficient to convey all the necessary information about the progress of the patient although the mean frequency comes very close to it.

The mean frequency is of course a rather simple and non-specific descriptor of something as complex as an EEG signal but it has distinct advantages in being intuitively meaningful to clinicians and correlates remarkably well with expectations from the clinical state. It has found ready acceptance in clinical practice where the more accurate but complex frequency spectrum or even the abbreviated spectrum from broad band analogue filters has not. It is furthermore, a parameter which is easy to compute and lends itself to implementation in relatively simple stand alone monitoring devices.

For simplicity the expression for mean frequency for a discrete spectrum, obtained by taking the Fourier Transform of the signal is:

For an input signal V(t) with an amplitude spectrum given by A(f) for f=1, 2, 3, ...N

$$MF = \frac{\sum_{f=L}^{U} f \cdot A(f)}{\sum_{f=L}^{U} A(f)}$$

Where U and L are the upper and lower harmonics, respectively, defining the pass band of interest.

The continuous equivalent of this function may be implemented using analogue components as illustrated in figure 3. A full description will appear elsewhere (Quilter et al, in press). The input signal is fed through a linear weighting filter after being normalized by a voltage controlled amplifier circuit. The effect of this filter is to produce an output voltage which is proportional to frequency. The output of this filter is rectified and integrated (T.C. 3 or 10 secs) to give the mean frequency.

A picture of the monitor is shown in Fig. 4. Input is from two active electrodes plus an earth into a small headbox. Input impedance is 4 megaohms. Output is in the form of two digital displays of mean frequency and mean amplitude and a two letter status indicator showing open circuit (OC) short circuit (SC) conditions of the electrodes, or HF (high frequency artefact) or LF (low frequency artefact) conditions detected by overflow outside the 1-25 Hz pass band which would invalidate the measured parameters.

DFAM I

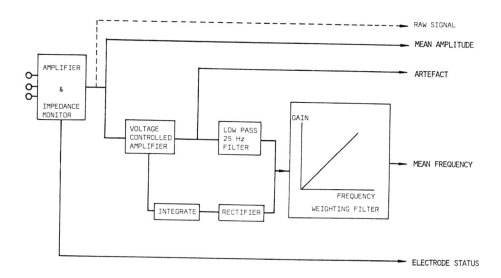

Fig. 3 Block diagram of digital mean frequency and amplitude monitor (DFAM) showing the key filter which outputs a voltage proportional to frequency. Mean amplitude is simply the rectified and integrated raw signal. Both M.F. and M.A. are smoothed by output time constants of 3 or 10 seconds (switchable).

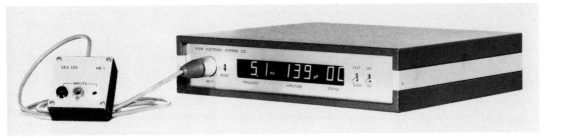

Fig. 4 Physical appearance of the monitor. The digital readout is two figures for mean frequency, three for mean amplitude and H, L, S.C. or O.C., for electrode and input status. The switch on the right selects 3 or 10 second smoothing time constant. (The figures displayed are for illustration only).

A permanent record may be held from chart or tape outputs from the rear of the machine together with the amplified signal. The state of the status displays is also output (No display = valid recording conditions).

There are a few features of the device which deserve particular mention:

Input: The normal method of using a.c. capacitive coupling components to remove the effects of standing skin/electrode potentials, has been changed. Instead a pseudo-d.c. amplifier is used which automatically offsets any d.c. component in the input signal (Quilter et al, in press). The dynamic range is 1-500 μV.

Electrode Monitoring: The impedance between the active electrodes is continuously monitored by injecting 1KHz sine wave signal and measuring the current flowing between the electrodes at this frequency. If the impedance drops below predefined level (1Kohm) the status indicator shows SC (short circuit). If the impedance rises above a predefined level (50 Kohm) the status indicator shows OC (open circuit). The patient electrodes interface, as in all direct monitoring procedures, is a critical factor to success and the necessity for such continuous automatic testing cannot be overemphasised.

Raw Signal Output: For the parameter being displayed to be validated it is essential that the raw EEG signal can be periodically observed. A high level signal output has been provided for display on an oscilloscope or chart recorder, or tape storage.

Chart Recorder Output: A modified two channel chart recorder can be incorporated with the monitor. The recorder has two speeds, a slow speed chosen to be in the range 1mm/min to 30mm/min and a fast speed of 24 mm/sec. The recorder is modified such that when it is in the slow speed position it displays the mean frequency and mean amplitude values. In the fast position the channel normally used to display the mean amplitude is used instead to write out the raw signal. This allows a permanent record of the measured parameters to be interspersed with a sample from the EEG record occuring at that time (Fig. 5). The recorder also indicates the type of any status artefact by full scale pen deflections on upper (electrode SC or OC) or lower (L and H frequency artefact) channels.

Some examples of the results obtained with EEG signals from patients in various degrees of liver failure are illustrated in Fig. 6 together with computer generated spectral energies for the same signals for comparison. The monitor when tested with pure sine wave inputs in one or combinations of frequencies, gives results well within the design parameters of better than 5%.

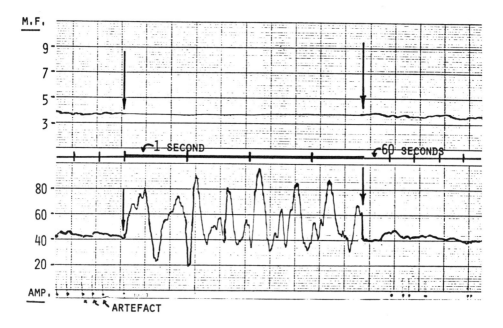

Fig. 5 An example of chart output showing a mean frequency (M.F.) of 3.8 Hz and mean amplitude (M.A.) of ± 44 µV interrupted by a sample of the raw record between arrows. Note different time scales and artefact blips.

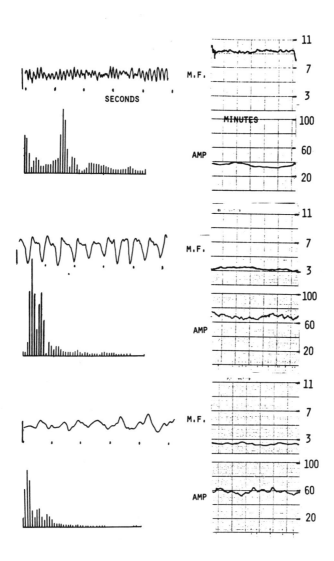

Fig. 6 The illustration shows the EEG of three different stages of coma on the left, the spectral energy from 0-25 Hz in 0.5 Hz steps below, and 6 minute samples of the monitor output for each record on the right. The spectra show a characteristic 'shift to the left' which is reflected in the falling mean frequency. (Calibration bar for EEG trace=100 μV)

As has been mentioned, the clinical condition of liver failure is probably a multifactor phenomenon. It is possible, however, to reproduce a similar series of clinical changes in experimental animals using substances thought to be the cause of the brain disturbances associated with liver failure. An example is shown in Fig. 7 which illustrates the dose/response relationship of the EEG in the rabbit to injection of a short chain fatty acid (Valearic). Of course it is not possible to follow patients through a similar time course from normal to coma and death or recovery since they are invariably in coma or precoma when first admitted, but by pooling the results from many such patients and assuming that the recovery function is the reverse of deterioration (which seems to be true), we can plot out a diagram of the sequence of the EEG changes in terms of the parameters measured in relation to the clinical grade, as in Fig. 8.

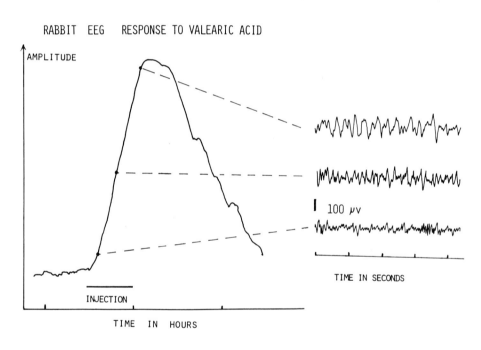

Fig. 7 EEG dose/response relations in rabbit given valearic acid to illustrate how quantification of the EEG can define such relations Examples of EEG are shown on the right. The computer generated curve is derived from the changes in the 1-3 Hz components of the EEG with time. (Accumulation of short chain fatty acids is believed to be a factor in producing liver coma. Experiments conducted at The Royal Post Graduate Hospital (Dr. D. A. Calne and colleagues) EEG data processing at Royal Free Hospital).

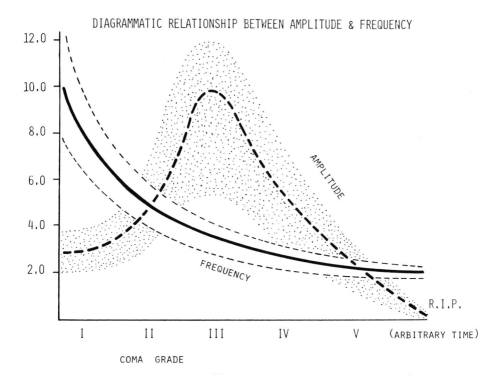

Fig. 8 Diagrammatic representation of the apparent course of the M.F. and M.A. measurements from normal on the left to death in liver coma on the right. The curves represent interpolations from many different subjects plotted against an arbitrary linear time course of degree of clinical coma, I-V. The dashed and dotted outlines indicate the order of variance expected across subjects. Figures on the left can be read as mean frequency or tens of microvolts.

It must be emphasised that although based on a fairly considerable experience, the diagram is speculative. The mean frequency appears to fall in an approximately exponential way from a normal value of about 10 Hz with a fairly high variance across subjects to a low of about 2Hz, where it remains till death. Mean amplitude on the other hand, which has a much higher variance across subjects, although a particular subject will follow the pattern of the curve with high predictability, rapidly rises to a peak amplitude corresponding to a mean frequency of about 3.5 then falls to zero with death. With increasing degrees of coma, the variance in a subject and across subjects decreases quite markedly as suggested in the diagram.

In practice, patients whose EEG's fall on the right hand side of the figure, particularly coma grades iv and v, (M.F.2.5 with falling amplitude) have a very poor prognosis and rarely survive. The EEG changes in liver failure are paralleled in a number of other conditions, kidney failure, anaesthesia and cerebral anoxic states for example, and thus equally amenable to monitoring with the same parameters but different dose response relationships.

Our experience has been of ready acceptance of this form of monitoring in a clinical situation which is at best complex and difficult.

REFERENCES

Kennedy, J., Parbhoo, S.P., MacGillivray, B., Sherlock, S. (1973). Effect of Extracorporeal liver perfusion on the Electroencephalogram of patients in coma due to acute liver failure, Quart. J. Med., 42:549-561.

Lunzer, M. (1975). Encephalopathy in liver disease, Brit. J. Hosp. Med., 13:33-44.

MacGillivray, B. (1969). An EEG monitor incorporating simple pattern recognition, J. Physiol. (Lond). 201. 65-67P.

MacGillivray, B. (1975). The EEG in liver disease:in Handbook of Electroencephalography and clinical Neurophysiology, Vol.15 Part C (in press).

THE USE OF EEG TELEMETRY AND VIDEORECORDING IN THE DIFFERENTIAL

DIAGNOSIS OF FITS

    A.N. Bowden

    University Department of Clinical Neurology

    The National Hospital, Queen Square, London

    Over the last 3 years a research programme at the National Hospital, supported by a grant from the DHSS has had the following aims: 1) to set up facilities for the close observation of patients with their electroencephalograms (EEGs) over relatively long periods of time; 2) to assess the value of these in the investigation of patients with epilepsy or suspected epilepsy, with emphasis on those patients whose diagnosis or treatment presented problems. This has been a combined enterprise involving Professor R.W. Gilliatt, Dr. R.G. Willison and myself from the University Department of Clinical Neurology, Dr. W.A. Cobb from the Hospital Department of Clinical Neurophysiology, Mr. P. Fitch (project engineer), and Mrs. Jacobson and Miss Short (recordists).

    Patients are observed in a room on the ward. 8 channels of EEG are obtained by telemetry using a small radiotransmitter weighing about 250 G. pinned to the patient's shirt. The receiver and demodulator are in the same room. Separate TV cameras cover the patient and a 4-channel EEG display on a memory monitor; the pictures from both are mixed so that each occupies half the viewing screen of a TV monitor. The numerical display of a real time code is also mixed into the TV picture. Signals are passed through cable to a basement laboratory 3 floors below the ward where recordings are made. The 8 EEG channels are recorded on a 14-channel FM tape-recorder, with spare channels for real time code and for audio from a microphone in the observation room. The mixed TV signal is recorded on videotape, which also has an audio channel. Observation sessions have usually lasted several hours and include a meal and nap. Subsequently EEG tapes and videotapes are searched for clinical attacks and interictal EEG abnormalities.

In practice we have gained far more information from monitoring patients in this way than from conventional EEG recording and ward observation. The method has been particularly valuable in deciding whether attacks are epileptic or not, whether epileptic attacks are associated with generalised or focal EEG discharge, whether there are specific triggers for a patient's attacks, and in following the effects of anticonvulsant drugs. In the differential diagnosis of fits it is helpful to record clinical attacks and any interictal epileptic activity in the EEG. We have obtained a much higher yield of both from long recordings than from routine 20 minute EEG recordings in the hospital EEG department (Tables 1 and 2). Ciné films can be made from the videotapes for teaching purposes.

A diagram of the monitoring system and photograph of the TV display can be found in Proceedings of the Royal Society of Medicine, 68, 246-248 (1975).

Table 1. Epileptic and non-epileptic clinical attacks obtained during long recordings with telemetry and TV monitoring (average duration 300 mins.) compared with routine EEG recordings in the Hospital EEG Department (average duration 20 mins.).

	Total No. of patients studied	No. of patients in whom clinical attacks recorded	
		Epileptic	Non-epileptic
Long recording	109	38	19
Routine recording	109	13	4

Table 2. Number of epileptic patients with epileptic activity in the EEG in long recordings compared with routine recordings.

	Total No. of epileptic patients studied	No. of patients with epileptic activity in EEG
Long recording	75	66
Routine recording	75	31

HAEMODYNAMIC ASSESSMENT BY TRANSCUTANEOUS AORTOVELOGRAPHY IN INTENSIVE THERAPY

Judith Beardshaw
Brompton Hospital, London, S.W.3

Gillian C. Hanson
Whipps Cross Hospital, London, E.11

Transcutaneous aortovelography, or T.A.V., is a noninvasive technique for measuring instantaneous aortic blood velocity, which serves as an index of left ventricular output.

The measurement is based on the Doppler principle and uses an ultrasonic beam at 2MHz. This energy is backscattered by red cells moving round the aortic arch with a frequency shift which is proportional to the blood velocity.

The Doppler equation may be written as :

$$\Delta f = \frac{2f \cdot V}{C} \text{ Cosine } \theta$$

where f = 2MHz, the frequency of the emitted beam,

V is the velocity of the moving target (aortic bloodstream)

C is the velocity of ultrasound at 2MHz through intervening tissue, about 1.55×10^3 M/sec.

θ is the angle between the emitted beam and the direction of blood flow

so that $\Delta f = 25.8 \, V \cdot \cos \theta$ Hz.

When θ is less than $26°$, $\cos \theta$ has a value of 0.9 to 1.0, so that V calculated from the equation assuming an angle of $0°$ is accurate to within 10%.

There is no need for any calibration when velocities are

calculated in this way from measured frequency shifts.

The Doppler-shifted frequencies are subjected to on-line spectral analysis so that the instrument is direction resolving and the highest negative Doppler shifts, resulting from mainstream receding flow in the aortic arch, are easily extracted and displayed on a paper write-out (Fig. 1).

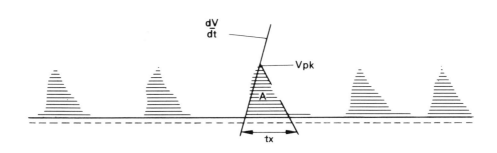

Fig. 1

Method

The patient lies supine and the transducer is applied to the suprasternal notch using an ultrasonic coupling gel. The direction of the transducer is adjusted until the characteristic Doppler sounds of arterial blood flow are heard on the loudspeaker. The recorder is then switched on and the transducer is again aimed to display a record containing the highest velocities and a clear signal with a sharp outline at a standard intensity. The transducer is usually pointing downwards and to the left in order to align the ultrasonic beam with blood flow to the transverse arch of the aorta.

The controls which are constantly used during recording - record on/off, display intensity and an event marker - are on a small, handheld, remote control box, so that one person can conveniently operate the instrument.

Interpretation

The outline of the aortic blood velocity signal consists of the highest Doppler shifts received. Even if other vessels are within the beam, no vessel in this area normally contains receding blood flowing with such high velocities in a direction so closely aligned with the beam. Venous signals are usually readily distinguishable as they contain relatively low Doppler shifts and by their diastolic timing.

To compare different flow rates, the aortic cross sectional area and velocity profile must remain reasonably constant from one observation to the next.

The major factors which make calculation of absolute values of cardiac output from the mean aortic velocity unreliable include:

1. the measurement is made at the transverse aortic arch, so that it must be corrected for blood which has already left the aorta to supply the heart, head and neck, back and upper limbs.
2. calculation of the aortic cross section is not reliable.
3. quantitative interpretation is based on the assumption that the aortic velocity profile is flat.

When respiratory modulation is present, the record should be analysed over an integral number of respiratory cycles.

In most patients, we found that visual assessment of the record gave useful sequential information: the height of the trace gave the peak velocity, the length gave ejection time, and the area under the velocity outline gave an index of stroke volume. Traces are now being analysed quantitatively to facilitate the interpretation of less obvious waveform changes and for documentation and statistical purposes.

Hand analysis of traces (Fig. 2)

A number of parameters can be defined by fitting straight lines to the leading and trailing edges of the complex. These include V_{xp}, the extrapolated peak velocity. The area, A, of the complex is related to stroke volume and is approximated by $A = \frac{1}{2} V_{xp} . t$, where t is the extrapolated ejection time. $\bar{V}$ is the time-averaged mean velocity of blood entering the descending aorta and is given by -

$$\bar{V} = \frac{A}{T}$$ where T is the period of the cardiac cycle.

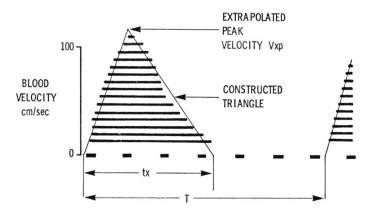

Fig. 2. Hand Analysis of Flow Velocities

Comparison with other cardiac output measurements

Comparative measurements have been performed by Dr. Raftery and Dr. Sequeira at Northwick Park Hospital, Harrow, Middlesex. Cardiac output was measured in 20 patients by the indicator dilution technique at rest and during atrial pacing at rates up to 160 per minute. Good proportionality was found with T.A.V. measurement, but the agreement with absolute values of cardiac output was too poor for clinical use. The good proportionality suggests that T.A.V. may be used to compare different flow rates in one patient.

Clinical experience

Experience has been gained in a busy Intensive Therapy Unit serving approximately 1500 acute beds. During the first four months we took traces from most patients admitted to the Intensive Therapy Unit and during the next four months we made a critical appraisal of T.A.V.'s possible use.

Preliminary work with Mr. H. Light, Dr. Judith Beardshaw and co-workers has been undertaken to assess the consistency of data obtained as described above, with five observers and eleven volunteer 'normal' subjects, and ten healthy children. The coefficients of variation were as follows :

Repeat recordings by:	Vxp	Area	V̄
Same observer	3.9%	6.0%	6.4%
Different observers	4.6%	7.0%	7.4%

The consistency found indicates that changes exceeding 10% should be observable with greater than 90% confidence.

CONDITIONS STUDIED

Myocardial Infarction

Most patients admitted to the Intensive Therapy Unit with myocardial infarction had associated complications such as left ventricular failure or cardiac dysrhythmias. T.A.V., in conjunction with other observations, may give an indication of the cardiovascular response to drugs, thereby facilitating patient management. Sequential T.A.V. traces at different endocardial pacing rates may enable the pacing rate to be set at optimum left ventricular output.

Shock

The management of the shocked, critically ill patient can be complex; clinical examination alone is often inadequate.

The management of hypovolaemic shock in a young patient with overt blood loss rarely presents difficulty. The situation becomes more complex when there is no evidence of blood volume loss, cardiac or renal failure is suspected and sepsis is a possibility. In such circumstances, other observations should be made to facilitate patient management.

In hypovolaemic shock, central venous pressure monitoring in conjunction with observations of pulse rate, blood pressure and hourly urine output is generally adequate. In severe shock, even the placement of a central venous catheter may be difficult. T.A.V. traces taken on patients with hypovolaemic shock show low peak velocities associated with low mean velocities.

Figure 3 shows serial changes in a patient admitted with severe hypovolaemic shock.

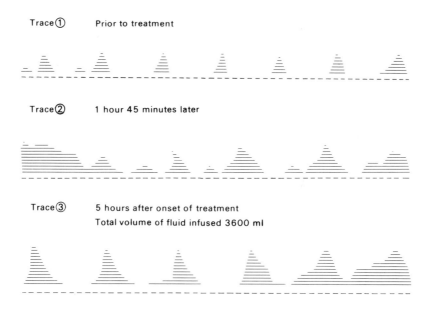

Fig.3. Hypovolaemic shock

Figure 4 shows the various observations taken during treatment of the shocked state. The systolic B.P. was unrecordable on admission and the mean velocity recorded on the T.A.V. trace was extremely low. Fluid therapy was commenced on the basis of these findings and evidence of extensive fluid loss over the previous week. C.V.P. readings were not available for a further hour.

Increasing volumes of fluid were then given; the central venous pressure and blood pressure steadily rose - this was associated with an increased mean velocity showed by T.A.V., and urine output. The skin-core temperature difference also decreased as peripheral perfusion improved with fluid volume replacement.

T.A.V. may prove valuable in the therapeutic management of patients suffering from an overdose of drugs. The following traces are taken from a patient suffering from a severe amylobarbitone overdose (Table 5).

HAEMODYNAMIC ASSESSMENT IN INTENSIVE THERAPY

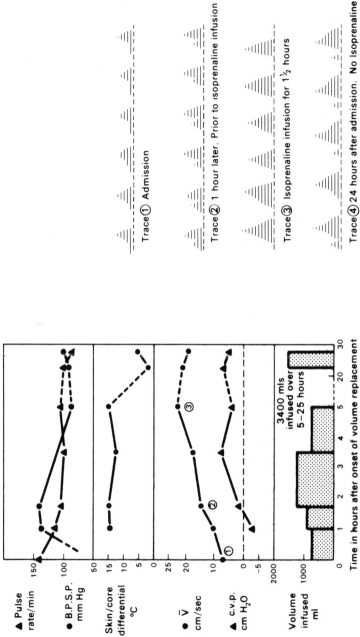

Fig. 4. Graph of progress in hypovolaemic shock

Fig. 5. Amylobarbitone overdose

Figure 6 shows the various parameters recorded. At the time of admission, the central venous pressure was high, the pulse rate was 150/minute, and the B.P. unrecordable. The mean velocity was low. These findings were consistent with a low cardiac output state presumably secondary to the myocardial suppressant effect of amylobarbitone. In view of the gross peripheral vasoconstriction and low output state, an isoprenaline infusion was started. This was followed by a fall in the central venous pressure, little increase in pulse rate and a dramatic increase in mean velocity shown by T.A.V. The drip rate of the isoprenaline infusion was regulated so that the pulse rate was maintained at less than 120/minute with an increased but submaximal mean velocity.

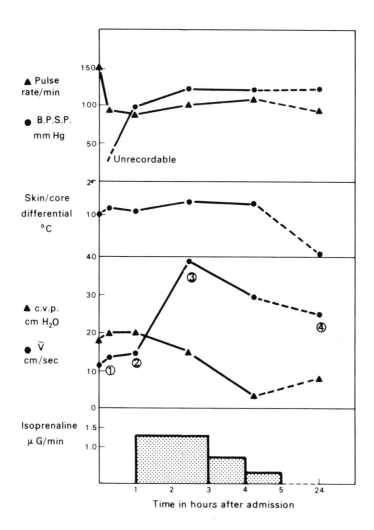

Fig.6. Graph of progress in a patient with amylobarbitone overdose

CONCLUSION

Over the last eight months, the technique of T.A.V. has been used (in conjunction with other conventional techniques) for the assessment of cardiovascular function in critically ill patients.

T.A.V. has the advantage over many other techniques for assessment of L.V. output in being noninvasive, consistent and generally convenient. Traces cannot be obtained in approximately 10% of patients, most of whom have tracheostomies.

Sequential traces can be taken with moderate ease and little patient discomfort. Pilot evaluation suggests that this technique provides useful information regarding cardiovascular status and serial traces may give a guide to progress and response to therapy.

DESIGN PRINCIPLES OF THE E.M.I. SCANNER

G. N. Hounsfield

E.M.I. Research Laboratories

Hayes, Middlesex

All are familiar with the shortcomings of the conventional X-ray techniques in attempting to display a two-dimensional picture (see Fig. 1) of a three-dimensional object. Also we are aware of their insensitivity to the differentiation between various forms of soft tissue. Nor do these techniques provide a means of measuring in any quantitative way, the density of the substances viewed. Computerised tomography is a new technique which successfully overcomes all of these limitations.

What, then, is computerised tomography? It is a technique for making visible the inside of an object by focusing attention upon a series of contiguous thin slices taken through it (see Fig.2). This provides total three-dimensional information. The system is approximately 100 times more sensitive than conventional X-ray techniques in differentiating various tissues, as it fully utilizes all the information that can be obtained from the emerging X-rays. Moreover, the densities of the tissues displayed within the slice can be quantified.

How, then, in practical terms, is the technique applied? Let us take, for example, its application to the human head. Fig. 3

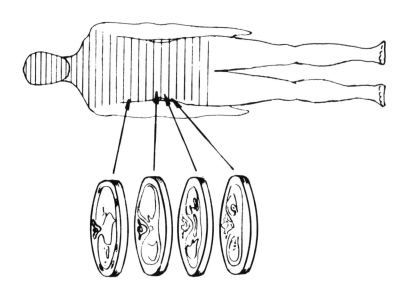

Fig. 2 COMPUTERIZED TOMOGRAPHY

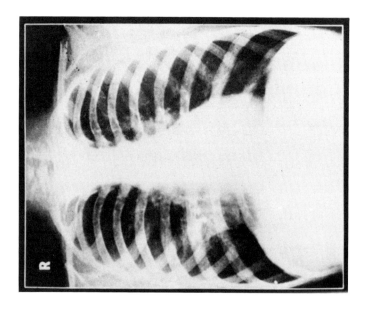

Fig. 1

DESIGN PRINCIPLES OF THE E.M.I. SCANNER

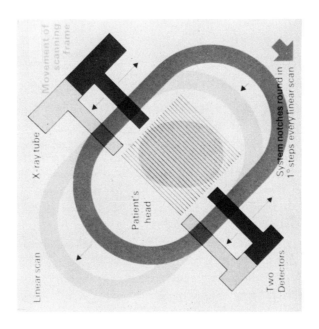

Fig. 4

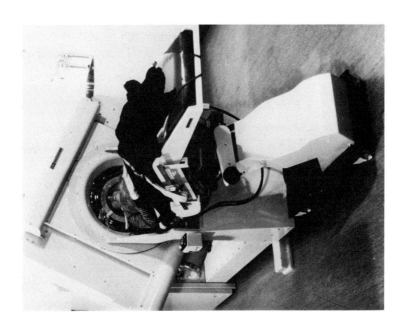

Fig. 3

is a picture of the E.M.I. Brain scanner and a patient about to be examined.

The patient is scanned by a narrow collimated beam of X-rays. The X-ray tube, detectors and collimators are fixed to a common frame, as shown (Fig. 4). Those rays which pass through the head are detected by collimated sensing devices which always point towards the X-ray source. Both X-ray source and detectors scan across the patient's head linearly, taking 240 readings of transmission through the head, as shown in SCAN ONE on the scanning sequence diagram (see Fig. 5). At the end of the scan, the scanning system is rotated 1 degree and the process is repeated as shown in SCANS TWO and THREE. This procedure continues for 180 scans, when 42,000 readings will have been taken by each detector in order to produce a picture of one single slice of the head (see Fig. 6). The right hand picture shows a large tumor bottom right. These readings are processed by a computer which mathematically reconstructs a picture of the absorption coefficient of the various substances within the slice. These can either be shown on a picture as tone gradients or be printed out in numerical values (see Fig. 7).

The numerical values are extremely accurate readings of absorption coefficient, measured to $\frac{1}{2}\%$ with respect to tissues.

Some idea of the scale of accuracy of the system can be demonstrated by the chart shown (Fig. 8). It can be seen that the absorption coefficient of fat is 10% less than that of water, and that of tissue, on average, is approximately 3% greater than that of water. Variation of tissue absorption found in the head including the ventricles covers a 4% range. The picture brightness and contrast can be adjusted so that this 4% range or "window" covers full black to peak white. The height of this "window" can also be adjusted to the level of any material which may be required to be viewed.

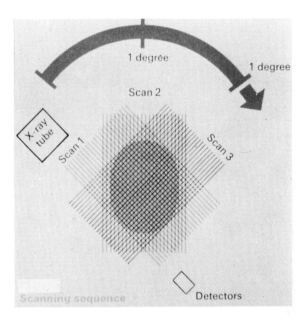

Fig. 5

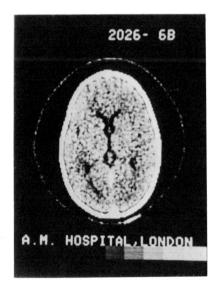 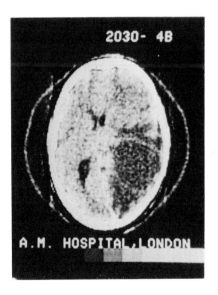

Fig. 6

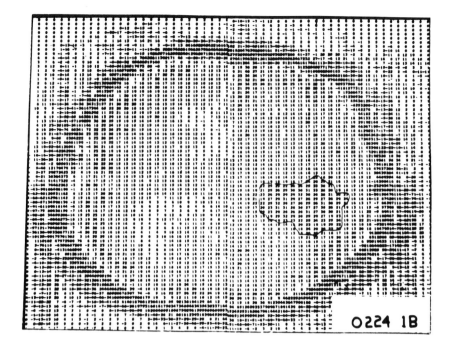

Fig. 7

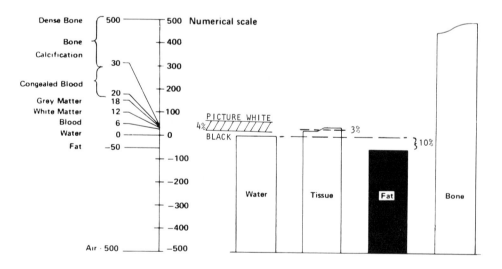

Fig. 8

CT techniques have, so far, been mainly restricted to the head and on the whole the results have been successful. But it was obvious, even from early days, that this technique might also be an excellent diagnostic tool for use on the body.

In designing a machine for body scanning, a number of additional factors needed to be considered, and these created a number of additional problems beyond those of brain scanning. However, we believe that these problems have now largely been overcome; a body machine has now been built at EMI Research Laboratories and is now undergoing trials at Northwick Park Hospital. The first picture that was produced by the machine in the laboratory (Fig. 9) is a picture of a slice taken through the abdomen.

In the larger and more complex area of the abdomen, it is necessary to obtain information about a number of different organs, some of which will occupy only a small area in the field of view. It is likely that much diagnostic information can be gained from studying the shape or displacement of these organs, which is generally emphasised by the outlining fat around them. This requires greater clarity than is normally called for from the brain machine. One important requirement, therefore, is for greater definition. The picture you see is displayed on a 320 x 320 matrix.

Another problem arises from the fact that the average torso is approximately 13" in diameter, in contrast to the brain's maximum diameter of 9". This increased length of path along which X-rays have to travel considerably reduces the number of photons arriving at the detectors. The effect of this, combined with the effect of seeking better definition as previously mentioned, is to increase the amplitude of the grain on a body picture by approximately a factor of five over that of a brain picture. This grain would tend to obscure the fine variations among tissues.

This is compensated to a certain extent by the fact that the body, unlike the head, contains a great deal of fat in and around the organs, which locates and outlines them. In the case of some tumor tissues, however, the grain amplitude may be so great as to obscure them unless an increased X-ray dose is given or a contrast medium is used. I should make it clear that in none of the pictures in this article has an increased X-ray dose been given to the patient to reduce the grain on this picture. Nor has a contrast medium been used. It should be noted also that because CT is a more sensitive process than conventional X-ray, it is capable of detecting very much smaller quantities of contrast media and for this reason may be possible to highlight various organs very successfully. The pictures shown (Figs. 10-14) are taken with a relatively small X-ray dose, 2-3 rads. An increased dose would improve resolution.

Fig. 10 is a picture taken through the kidney. If a very small amount of contrast media had been used in taking this scan, the kidneys would have shown up very much lighter in tone, and their details would have been highlighted with greater selectivity.

Fig. 11 is a slice two centimetres higher than Fig. 10 and reveals the pancreas clearly (arrowed). This is the first time the pancreas has been seen by means of X-rays. It is normally undetectable by conventional methods.

Fig. 12, approximately two centimetres higher than Fig. 11, reveals the liver and spleen. It is hoped that tumours on the liver may be visible without the aid of contrast media. This is yet to be ascertained from clinical trials.

Fig. 13 shows the lungs, which in common with some other organs, notably the heart, are in constant movement, which could cause considerable streaking and blurring on the picture. The

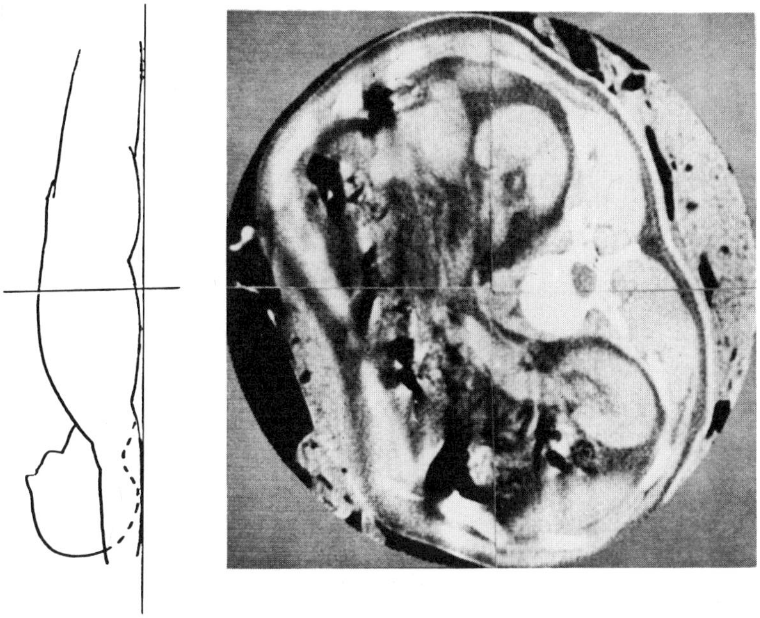

DESIGN PRINCIPLES OF THE E.M.I. SCANNER 127

Fig. 10

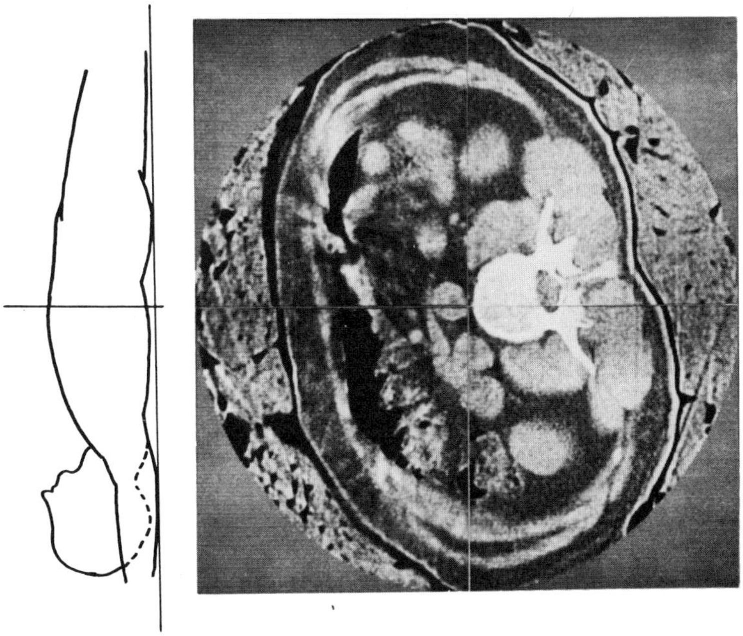

Fig. 9

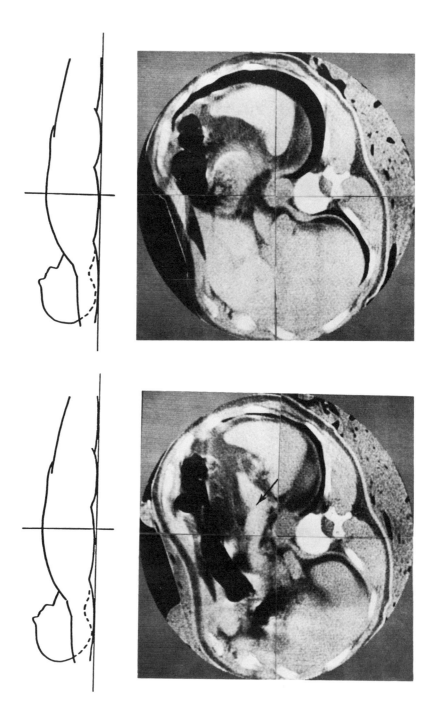

Fig. 12

Fig. 11

DESIGN PRINCIPLES OF THE E.M.I. SCANNER

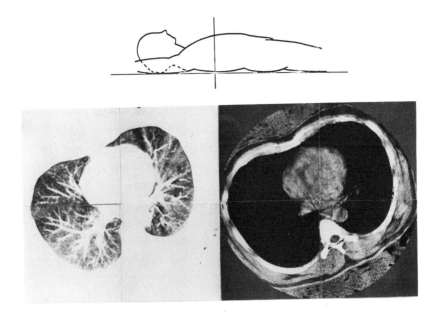

Fig. 13

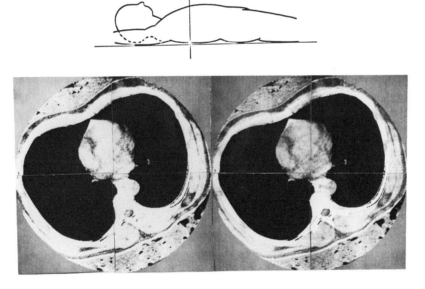

Fig. 14

picture shown is taken of the lungs and heart with a scanning time of twenty seconds, during which time a patient is capable of holding his breath without undue difficulty. This reduces movement to an acceptable level.

It can be seen from Fig. 14 that the problem of picture grain does not arise in the case of a scan across the heart and lungs. Due to the large volume of air, in the chest, a considerably greater number of photons are able to reach the detectors. The spinal cord can also be seen.

The pictures shown were taken in the laboratories of our EMI staff. It may be reasonably supposed that the full capabilities of the body machine can only be assessed after studies on patient cases have been made during the clinical trials that are in process at Northwick Park. Nevertheless, it seems clear that in CT we have a very powerful means at our disposal for enormously extending the diagnostic capabilities of X-ray techniques.

PRACTICAL EXPERIENCE WITH THE EMI SCANNER

J. GAWLER

THE NATIONAL HOSPITAL FOR NERVOUS DISEASES

QUEEN SQUARE, LONDON W.C.1 ENGLAND

Until the advent of computer assisted x-ray tomography the fundamental techniques used in x-ray examination had not changed since their introduction by Röentgen nearly eighty years ago. Two inherent difficulties have limited the conventional radiograph. First, the resolution of structures is possible only when they differ quite markedly in their capacity to absorb x-rays (thus bone can be distinguished from soft tissue but individual soft tissue structures are difficult to define) and second, even with conventional tomography, all structures in the long axis of an x-ray beam are superimposed on the radiograph. A plain x-ray of the head will display the bones of the skull, but will not resolve the brain or the fluid filled chambers which lie within it. Information about the intracranial content can be obtained from conventional x-ray techniques only with the aid of artificial contrast media. Thus, the introduction of air or an iodine containing fluid into the cerebral ventricles or subarachnoid space allows these structures to be seen, and similarly, contrast media can be injected into the blood vessels of the brain to give an image of the vascular tree. Such contrast procedures (encephalography or angiography) have been the only reliable means of defining many structural lesions, such as tumour or haemorrhage, within the skull. They require however, the patient's admission to hospital, often a general anaesthetic and all carry a small but quite definite risk in terms of both morbidity and mortality.

Computerized tomography yields information about structural brain disease which formerly could be obtained only from these elaborate investigations using contrast media. The EMI Scanner involves no discomfort, or risk for the patient, the result is available immediately and the x-ray exposure is no greater than that required for a single plain radiograph of the skull. The technique is sufficiently sensitive to measure the small difference in x-ray absorption between brain tissue and cerebrospinal fluid and in this way the ventricular system, subarachnoid cisterns and the cerebral or cerebellar sulci can be seen. Similarly cerebral grey and white matter may be contrasted because the density of the former is measurably greater than the latter. Structures, such as the basal ganglia or internal capsule, which could not be seen by conventional techniques, can now be identified by computerized tomography.

CEREBRAL ATROPHY AND HYDROCEPHALUS

Any enlargement of the ventricular system or widening of the cortical sulci is detected readily in patients with cerebral atrophy. In cerebellar atrophy the spaces between the folia are recognizably enlarged. Obstructive hydrocephalus is also easily diagnosed and can be distinguished from cerebral atrophy; often the responsible structural lesion can be seen at some point along the ventricular pathway. Comparative study between EMI Scans and pneumoencephalograms has shown an extremely high level of concordance between these two investigations in patients with cerebral atrophy or hydrocephalus.

Because ventricular size may be monitored so easily and without risk to the patient, the EMI Scanner is proving invaluable in the management of patients, such as those who have survived subarachnoid haemorrhage, who run a risk of developing hydrocephalus. Similarly patients whose hydrocephalus has been treated by shunting procedures can be serially assessed to determine the result of treatment or the presence of complications, such as a subdural haematoma.

CEREBRAL TUMOUR

Intracranial tumours may be detected on computerized scans in two ways. First, tumour tissue usually has a different density from the adjacent normal brain and the lesion itself can thus be delineated. Second, the presence of a mass may be indicated by its space occupying or obstructive effects on the ventricular system. The tissue density of vascular tumours may be measurably increased by scanning after an intravenous injection of an iodine containing contrast medium - (this procedure resembles that used in intravenous pyelography). The site, size and shape of a tumour may thus be discerned with great accuracy by this new technique, and it is possible to identify in addition local complications such as haemorrhage or oedema together with more distant complications like hydrocephalus.

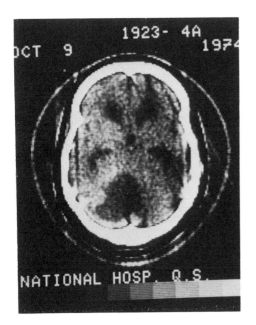 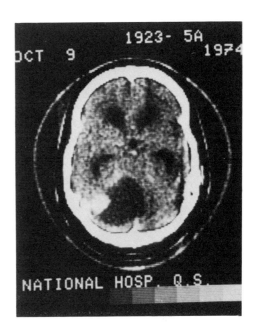

Fig. 1 Intracranial tumour. (4A before and 5A after an intravenous injection of Conray 420). Haemangioblastoma of the left cerebellar hemisphere. The site, size and shape of the tumour are well shown and its largely cystic nature is apparent. A vascular nodule (enhanced by iodine) is seen in the cyst wall on the left. Obstructive hydrocephalus is present.

The gross morphology of many tumours may be recognized and in this context the ability to resolve fluid filled cysts or the cystic components of a tumour preoperatively is particularly helpful. This information is of great value to the surgeon as he plans the operative approach and it cannot be obtained by any other investigation. The comparison of scans before and after the intravenous injection of iodine gives information about tumour blood supply and may disclose the presence of either a vascular capsule or tumour nodules in relation to a cystic or necrotic mass. The technique is so sensitive that it can detect the presence of calcification within tumours long before this could be seen by conventional methods. Fat is identified on computerized scans by its very low density and this finding is of significance in the preoperative recognition of those rare intracranial tumours, such as craniopharyngioma, cholesteatoma or teratoma, which contain lipid material. Lipomata of the corpus callosum also produce a characteristic appearance. It is important to realize that these morphological clues provided by computerized tomography are a valuable aid to the histological diagnosis of tumours.

The accuracy of the EMI Scanner in tumour diagnosis compares favourably with the conventional contrast investigations used in neuroradiology and is far superior to isotope brain scanning. The technique is also proving of great value in the early detection of tumour recurrence following treatment by surgery or radiotherapy.[1]

CEREBROVASCULAR DISEASE

Intracerebral or intraventricular haematomas can be diagnosed by computerized scanning because an accumulation of blood has a density greater than cerebral tissue.[2] Freshly shed blood increases slightly in density for the first 24 - 48 hours, presumably the result of coagulation and clot retraction, and then retains the same density for several days before falling as the haematoma is reabsorbed. Fresh haematomas are surrounded by a clear ring of low density, which represents extruded serum and cerebral oedema.

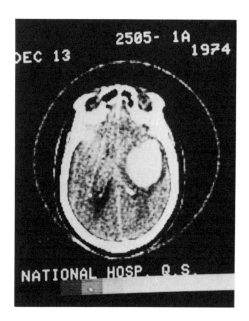 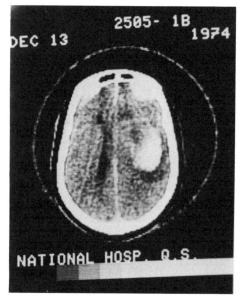

Fig. 2 Cerebral haemorrhage. A large intracerebral haematoma is present in the right temporal lobe. The high density clot is surrounded by diminished density due to cerebral oedema. The lateral ventricles are displaced to the left and the right lateral ventricle is attenuated by the mass.

The site and extent of a haematoma is shown more accurately by computerized scanning than by any other test, and only the scan can distinguish haematoma from oedema or recognize clotted blood within the ventricular system.

Cerebral infarction or oedema usually results in a reduction in tissue density and thus may always be distinguished from a fresh haematoma. With infarction a characteristic sequence of density change may be observed. The lesion becomes apparent within 24 - 48 hours, initially as a vague area of reduced density and increasing space occupying effect may be apparent at this stage. During the next 7 - 14 days the lesion becomes increasingly well defined, clearer at its edge, the density falls centrally and space occupying effect diminishes. Although some lesions seem to resolve, perhaps leaving slight ventricular enlargement or cortical atrophy as an indication of cerebral damage, the majority finally appear as well defined nonspace occupying low density zones or cysts.

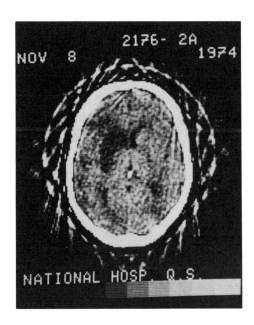 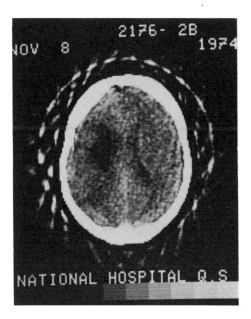

Fig. 3 Cerebral infarction. Scan undertaken one week after the sudden onset of right hemiplegia and aphasia. An extensive infarct lies deeply in the left cerebral hemisphere involving the basal ganglia and internal capsule.

The ability to rapidly and atraumatically distinguish haemorrhage from infarction or oedema is a tremendous advance not only for patients with stroke where it is now the radiological test of first choice, but also in the management of patients who have sustained serious head injury.

Subdural or extradural collections of blood can be located and blood may sometimes be seen in the subarachnoid cisterns of patients who have suffered subarachnoid haemorrhage. In patients shown to have multiple intracranial aneurysms by angiography, the detection of a small subarachnoid or intracerebral haematoma by computerized tomography may indicate which aneurysm has bled. When a patient's conscious level is falling after subarachnoid haemorrhage the ability to distinguish haematoma from oedema or infarction due to vascular spasm is invaluable.

CEREBRAL ABSCESS

Intracranial abscesses usually appear as extensive low density areas on computed scans. Intravenous contrast administration is most helpful in such patients for it is usually possible to display the vascular abscess capsule, to distinguish abscess from oedema and to define the number and distribution of loculi present.

INTRACRANIAL CALCIFICATION

Because the EMI Scanner can resolve calcified lesions before they become visible by conventional techniques, the method is of great value as a screening test in patients suspected of diseases, such as tuberose sclerosis, where widespread intracranial calcification develops. Several patients have been saved extensive investigation when focal intracranial calcification seen on the skull x-ray has raised the possibility of a tumour but computed scans have shown this to represent only a fraction of the widespread calcification caused by diseases such as toxoplasmosis.

ORBITAL DISEASE

Transverse tomography provides a new means of looking at the orbit. The low density of orbital fat provides a natural contrast against which the globe, optic nerve and extraocular muscles may be seen.

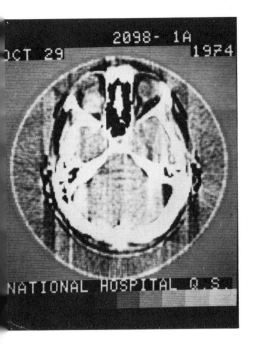 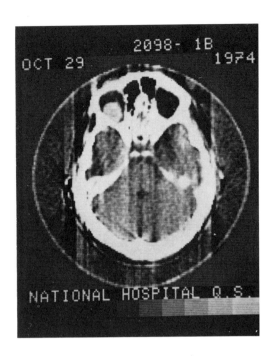

Fig. 4 Orbital tumour. Haemangioma of left orbit; in a patient with a ten year history of proptosis. The tumour was excised without further investigation. A normal optic nerve can be seen on the right in slice 1A.

Structural orbital lesions are readily shown tumour, granuloma or haematoma are all recognizable. Not only is the method proving extremely valuable for primary orbital disease but in addition it has given valuable evidence of the retrobulbar extension of tumours of the paranasal sinuses.[3]

CONCLUSION

When widely available, the EMI Scanner will dramatically alter the established investigative routine of patients suspected of having structural intracranial or orbital disease. An EMI Scan has become the radiological investigation of first choice for many neurological problems - intracranial and orbital tumour or abscess suspects, all strokes or head injuries and all those presenting with dementia. Furthermore, it is anticipated that computerized tomography will increase understanding of the nature and natural history of many brain diseases and provide a means of monitoring the effects of treatment. Conventional neuroradiological techniques will still be required to elucidate specific problems but the overall requirement for these has fallen dramatically at all centres already possessing an EMI Scanner. In this respect figures speak louder than words, and the number of pneumoencephalograms undertaken at the National Hospital has fallen from an average of 48 per month to 10 per month since the EMI Scan became available.

REFERENCES

1. Gawler J. du Boulay G.H. Bull J.W.D. Marshall J.
   Computer Assisted Tomography (EMI Scanner). Its Place in the Investigation of Suspected Intracranial Tumours.
   Lancet 1974, 2. 419-427.

2. Scott W.R. New P.F. et al. Computerized Axial Tomography of Intracranial and Intraventricular Haemorrhage.
   Radiology 1974, 112. 73-80.

3. Gawler J. Sanders M.D. et al. Computer Assisted Tomography in Orbital Disease.
   British Journal of Ophthalmology 1974, 58. 571-587.

VISUALLY EVOKED CORTICAL POTENTIALS IN NEUROLOGICAL DIAGNOSIS

A. M. Halliday

Medical Research Council, Institute of Neurology

National Hospital, Queen Square, London WC1

Pattern evoked response recording is a relatively new diagnostic technique which has shown itself to be particularly useful to the neurologist in the diagnosis of multiple sclerosis (Halliday, McDonald and Mushin, 1972, 1973a, 1976) and in the differentiation of organic and functional visual impairment (Halliday, 1972). The technique depends on measuring the small electrical potentials evoked by the arrival of a synchronous sensory volley at the cerebral cortex. When measured through the scalp, these potentials are only a few microvolts in size and they would be drowned in the much larger background electrical activity of the brain if one could not increase the sensitivity of the detection process. This can be done very effectively by adding a number of responses together and computing an average (Dawson, 1954).

The method is to sample the EEG for the short period after each stimulus during which the response is expected to occur, and to store the sample voltages in some sort of memory. Either analogue or digital methods may be used (Halliday and Pitman, 1965, Halliday, 1968). The stimulus - a sudden change in the pattern of light on a translucent screen viewed by the subject - is presented repeatedly (say, 100 times), and the corresponding samples are added to the accumulated sum of the previous responses. The result of this is that the stored response steadily grows in size in proportion to the number of stimuli delivered, but the background EEG, which is unrelated to the stimulus, will sometimes be positive and sometimes negative, and gradually averages itself out.

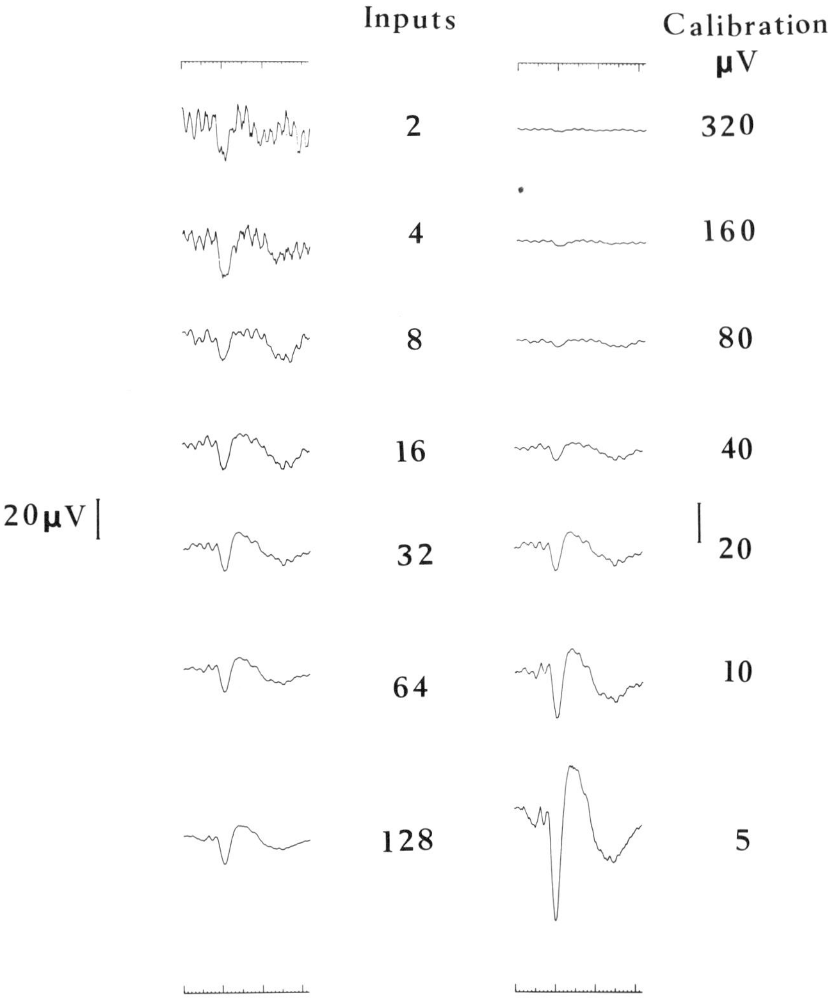

	Inputs		Calibration μV
	2		320
	4		160
	8		80
	16		40
20μV	32		20
	64		10
	128		5

Fig. 1. The growth of the summed occipital evoked responses during the presentation of an increasing number of pattern reversal stimuli (total indicated in central column) in a healthy subject, viewing a 32 degree stimulus field with both eyes open. In the left hand records a true average has been computed, illustrating the gradual disappearance of the background noise which obscures the response. In the right hand records is shown the more conventional display of a running sum, in which the summed response gradually grows out of the background. The average can be obtained from the running sum by adjusting the calibration for the number of input sweeps, as shown on the right.

The averaging process can therefore be regarded as a form of signal-noise discrimination. If one thinks of the responses as being of constant voltage (which, as a first approximation, they probably are), then the background noise level (or variance) is being reduced in proportion to the square root of the number of input waveforms, a process which can be seen in the left hand column of figure 1. In practice, rather than dividing the number of inputs to obtain the mean, one usually views the running sum and adjusts the calibration accordingly. The systematic response appears to grow in size in proportion to the number of inputs being added, while the background activity does not grow (see right hand column of figure 1).

The electrode recording the response on the scalp is placed as near as possible to the corresponding cortical receiving area. In the case of vision this is at the back of the head, and the maximal response to a visual stimulus is usually obtained with a mid-occipital electrode about 5 cms above the inion.

The averaging method demands a brief and accurately-timed stimulus, and traditionally visual evoked responses have usually been recorded using a flash stimulus, which can be easily provided from a gas discharge tube. However, we know from the work of Hubel and Wiesel (1962, 1968) that the neurones of the visual cortex are particularly interested in pattern stimuli, and are relatively insensitive to uniform illumination of their receptive field. This led us to investigate the averaged response to a reversing checkerboard pattern (Halliday and Michael, 1970, 1972; Michael and Halliday, 1971; Behrman, Halliday and McDonald, 1972).

In clinical testing, the patient is asked to fixate on a spot of light in the middle of a translucent screen, onto which a black and white checkerboard pattern is back-projected (Fig. 2). The pattern is reversed twice a second, so that the black squares become white and the white, black. The response to 200 such pattern reversals is averaged. The pattern stimulus is produced by projecting a checkerboard slide onto the screen by way of a mirror which can be rotated through a small angle to produce a rapid lateral displacement of the checkerboard through one square. Another way of producing the same kind of stimulus is with a television display (Arden, et al, 1976), but here the time taken to generate the pattern over the whole screen surface is appreciable (20 msec for a 50 c/s frame rate), and this may make accurate latency measurements of the response more difficult.

The occipital potential evoked by pattern reversal is rather stereotyped and contains a conveniently large and recognisable major positive component with a normal latency of about 100 msec. following the reversal. Typical normal responses from each eye of a healthy subject are shown on the left hand side of figure 3.

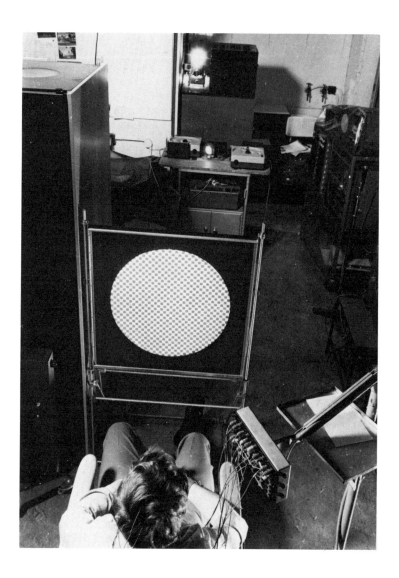

Fig. 2. General set-up for the pattern response test. The patient views a translucent screen onto the back of which a checkerboard pattern is projected. The pattern is reversed twice a second by rotating the small mirror via which it is projected onto the screen. The occipital electrodes and headboard connections can also be seen.

VISUALLY EVOKED CORTICAL POTENTIALS

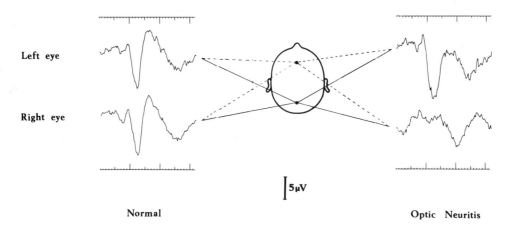

Fig. 3. Typical mid-occipital pattern evoked responses, recorded separately from each eye, in a healthy subject (left hand records) and in a patient, seen three weeks after an attack of acute unilateral optic neuritis in the right eye (right hand record). Note the reduced amplitude and delayed latency of the response from the affected eye. Time scale: 10, 50 and 100 msec.

The response from each eye is obtained in a separate run with the subject viewing the screen monocularly, the other eye being covered with an eye pad. The pair of responses shown on the right of figure 3 are from a patient recovering from an acute attack of optic neuritis in the right eye, recorded three weeks after onset. The response from the affected right eye is both delayed and reduced in amplitude, while the response from the unaffected left eye is very similar to those recorded in the healthy subject.

The latency of the occipital pattern response varies systematically with stimulus brightness (Halliday, McDonald and Mushin, 1973b) and is also affected by the speed of the pattern reversal (Halliday, McDonald and Mushin, 1973a). With a standardised stimulus, however, the latency of the major component varies over only a very small range in different individuals. Using a mirror stimulator capable of producing a complete pattern reversal within 10 msec, the mean latency for a group of 18 healthy subjects was 103.8 ± 4.3 msec (Halliday, McDonald and Mushin, 1973a), which is a similar latency to that produced by a pattern reversal effected by switching from one projector to another, using fast shutters (Halliday and Michael, 1970). In the group of healthy young adults tested, all the responses fell within a range of 20 msec. This allows one to set up a criterion for a pathologically delayed response with virtually no danger of any false positive results being contributed by the healthy population. A suitable cut-off point, defining a delayed response, is a latency of more than 2½ standard deviations above the normal group mean, i.e. > 114.55 msec with this particular stimulus.

The latent period is partly taken up by retinal delays and partly by the time taken for the sensory volley to travel from the eye to the cortex. There may also be cortical delays as well. Because of the tight normal distribution of the latency, the test is very sensitive to any marked change in the conduction velocity in the afferent pathways. In demyelinating disease the optic nerve is very commonly the site of a plaque, and it has been shown experimentally that such an area of demyelination is associated with a delay in the conduction of the nerve impulses over the demyelinated segments (McDonald and Sears, 1970). In severe demyelination, transmission may fail altogether owing to conduction block, but in less severely affected fibres (and in the recovery stage following an acute attack) marked slowing of the normal conduction may be the most striking feature. The latency of the pattern evoked response is very sensitive to this conduction delay. In a series of 53 patients, recorded following an attack of optic neuritis, all except three had a latency definitely beyond the normal range (Halliday, McDonald and Mushin, 1973b). The amplitude of the pattern response in the normal population is much more variable than the latency, and it is not possible to specify any normal limits which can be usefully employed to distinguish the normal from the pathological response. However, this is not to say that the amplitude change is not significant. Over the whole patient group, the amplitude is reduced following an attack of optic neuritis, paralleling the impairment of visual acuity, and recovers following an attack with the improving acuity level (Halliday, McDonald and Mushin, 1973b). The pathological increase in latency shows no such recovery and, once established, appears to persist indefinitely. The amplitude of the response from the two eyes is very similar in any individual, and amplitude differences recorded in the response from the two eyes in a single individual may be clinically significant even in an individual case, as in Fig. 3 and Fig. 4.

Figure 4 shows the pattern response recorded from a 24-year-old man four weeks after the onset of optic neuritis in the right eye. It can be seen that the large down-going positive component occurs at the normal latency in the response from the unaffected eye and that it is maximal in the midline channel. A very small response to the pattern reversal can be seen in the ERG recorded from peri-orbital electrodes positioned near the stimulated eye. In this patient visual acuity in the right eye

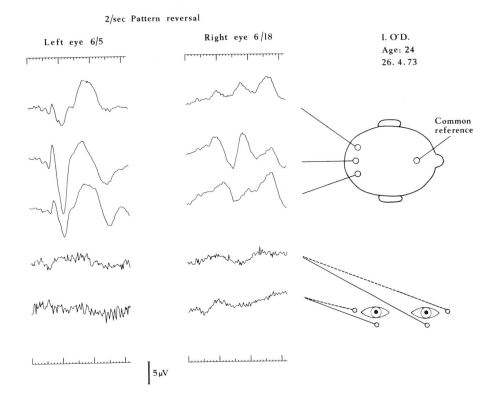

Fig. 4. Occipital response and ERG recorded from each eye of a patient recovering from right unilateral optic neuritis. Note the ERGs of similar waveform and latency from both affected and unaffected eyes, whereas the occipital response is delayed and reduced in amplitude in the affected eye. Time scale: 10, 50 and 100 msec.

had been reduced to counting fingers during the early acute phase of the attack, but it had improved to 6/18 at the time this record was taken four weeks later. The major positive component from the affected eye is clearly recognisable in the midline channel, but it is reduced in amplitude and markedly delayed in latency as compared with the left eye. The ERG pattern stimulus is, however, undelayed, and of very similar form to that from the left eye, emphasizing that the delay is taking place somewhere behind the eye, between the retina and the cortex.

Optic nerve plaques are extremely common in multiple

sclerosis. A definite history of retrobulbar neuritis is not unusual, but in many patients the clinician finds temporal pallor of the optic discs even where there is no history of any visual disturbance. The pattern response test has shown itself to be even more sensitive than fundoscopy in detecting clinically silent optic nerve lesions.

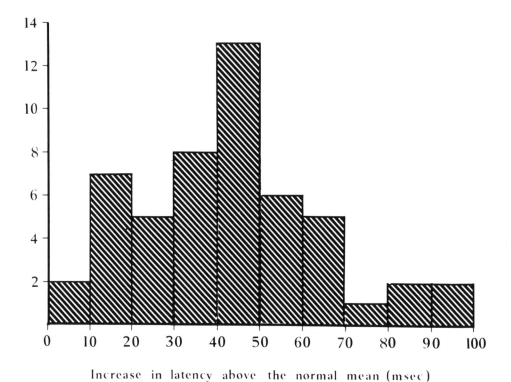

Fig. 5. Distribution of the observed delays in 51 patients with multiple sclerosis. Number of patients in each group indicated on the ordinate scale. Patients with a latency of more than 12 msec above the mean are outside the normal range and therefore pathologically delayed. Only two of these patients had latencies falling within the normal range.

Since the normal mean latency of the pattern response has such a small variance, the patient data can be expressed simply in terms of the increase in latency over the normal mean. Figure 5 shows the distribution of delays in 51 patients recorded by Halliday, McDonald and Mushin (1973a), all satisfying McAlpine's criteria for the diagnosis of multiple sclerosis (McAlpine, Lumsden and Acheson, 1972). The distribution of delays is very similar to that in the original series of young adult patients with acute unilateral optic neuritis (Halliday, McDonald and Mushin, 1972). The mean delay in the earlier series was 35 msec, while in this group of patients with multiple sclerosis it was 43.3 + 20.1 msec. The maximal delay was 100 msec in both series. Adopting an increase of more than 2½ times the standard deviation of the normal mean as the criterion of delay, two of the 51 patients with multiple sclerosis would be classified as within the normal latency range.

The 51 patients whose responses are included in figure 5 came from a total of 73 referred for suspected multiple sclerosis, the other 22 not having satisfied the diagnostic criteria laid down by McAlpine et al (1972). Only three of these 22 other cases had delayed responses. Thus there is both positive and negative evidence that the test is achieving a very high correlation with the diagnosis. The hit rate in this series in terms of the clinical criteria, is about 96%, and the test is picking up some delayed cases which the criteria failed to diagnose. The overall incidence of delays in the whole 73 referrals is just over 70% (see Table 1).

TABLE I

INCIDENCE OF DELAYED PATTERN RESPONSE IN
SUSPECTED MULTIPLE SCLEROSIS

	Number of cases	Number delayed
Multiple Sclerosis	51	49 (96%)
Other diagnosis or not yet diagnosed	22	3 (14%)
Total number referred	73	52 (71%)

TABLE II

INCIDENCE OF DELAYED PATTERN RESPONSE IN MULTIPLE SCLEROSIS PATIENTS WITH NEGATIVE VISUAL HISTORY AND NORMAL FUNDI

	Number of cases	Number delayed
Total number of patients with MS	51	49 (96%)
No history of optic neuritis	27 (53%)	25 (93%)
Normal optic discs	23 (45%)	21 (91%)
No history of optic neuritis and normal discs	14 (27%)	12 (86%)

In the group of 51 cases satisfying the criteria, we were surprised to find a high incidence of delays in those patients who had no history of any visual disturbance. More than half the patients fell into this group. The incidence of delayed responses in this sub-group fell only slightly, from 96 to 93% (Table II). The same was true of those patients who had no evidence of disc pallor on ophthalmoscopy; 91% of these had definitely delayed responses. The pattern response test therefore appears to be one of the most sensitive methods we have of detecting optic nerve damage. It is definitely more sensitive than any of the other clinically useful tests examined, including tests of colour vision and perimetry (Halliday, McDonald and Mushin, 1973a).

Multiple sclerosis is not the only cause of delayed responses, but it appears to be the most common, and in our own series over 90% of patients with this diagnosis had delays. The pattern response may be particularly useful as a screening test in the differential diagnosis of progressive spastic paraplegia. It is often difficult to differentiate between spinal cord compression and multiple sclerosis in patients who present with signs of a cord lesion, but have no objective evidence of a separate intracranial lesion. A delayed pattern response provides such evidence, and will often make it unnecessary to subject the patient to myelography.

In the first series of 27 cases referred because of progressive spastic paraplegia, we found 13 with delayed pattern evoked responses (Halliday, McDonald and Mushin, 1974). These

TABLE III

VEP IN PATIENTS WITH PROGRESSIVE SPASTIC PARAPLEGIA

	Number of cases referred	Abnormal VEP
Multiple Sclerosis	10	8
Cord Tumour	2	0
Cervical Spondylosis	2	0
Not yet diagnosed	13	5
Total number of cases	27	13

included eight of the 10 patients who could be diagnosed as suffering from multiple sclerosis on other grounds, and five undiagnosed cases. Four cases, who were shown on subsequent myelography to have either a cord tumour or cervical spondylosis, had normal responses.

Although it is particularly useful in the diagnosis of multiple sclerosis, the pattern evoked potential can also provide useful information for the neurologist or ophthalmologist in other conditions. Figure 6 shows the responses recorded in a 45-year-old woman, presenting with a seven months history of headaches and impaired vision in the right eye. She was first recorded in November 1972. The response from the right eye showed a major positivity of reduced amplitude, altered waveform and slightly delayed latency (Fig. 6). The response from the left eye at this time was within normal limits. Visual acuity was 6/9 in the right eye and 6/5 in the left. Six months later she was re-admitted for investigation and now had an altitudinal defect of the right lower half field extending into the upper field 10 degrees above the fixation point. Visual acuity was 6/6 in the left eye, but was reduced to the perception of hand movements in the right eye. The right optic disc was pale; the left disc appeared normal. By this time the pattern response from the right eye was completely abolished, and the response from the left eye was noticeably smaller and slightly broader than on the previous occasion. At this stage a carotid angiogram and a brain scan demonstrated a meningioma of the medial head of the lesser sphenoidal wing on the right, approximately 4 cms in diameter.

Shortly after this, the meningioma was removed at craniotomy, and she was recorded again five days post-operatively when visual acuity had improved to 6/60 in the right eye. In spite of this marginal improvement in vision, the pattern response from the right eye showed no appreciable recovery, while the response from the left eye was of larger amplitude than even the first pre-operative record, and the slight broadening of the major component, noticed pre-operatively, had disappeared. The acuity of the left eye had been normal throughout, which shows that the pattern response test is a rather sensitive one for detecting minimal impairment.

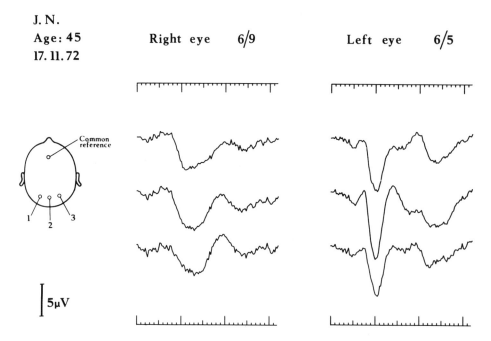

Fig. 6. Pattern evoked responses recorded in a then undiagnosed 45-year-old woman, with several months' history of headache and impaired vision in the right eye. Six months later, by which time visual acuity in the right eye was reduced to the perception of hand movements, a right sphenoidal wing meningioma was diagnosed radiologically and removed at operation.

In a series of 19 cases with compressive lesions of the anterior visual pathways we have found abnormal responses in 18, though not all were delayed (Halliday, McDonald and Mushin, 1975). It is likely that delay in the pattern response only occurs where there has been demyelination associated with compression.

Other conditions in which we have found delayed responses include some cases of hereditary spino-cerebellar ataxia and some congenital optic atrophies. Cappin and Nissim (1975) have recently reported delays in the steady state response to higher frequency pattern stimulation of the affected segments of the retina in glaucoma. Apart from delays, which appear to be associated with demyelination, the test may provide information which is useful in diagnosing retinopathies and in optic neuropathies associated with axonal degeneration of the visual fibres. In these cases it is mainly the amplitude, and sometimes also the waveform, of the response which is affected. The electroretinogram to flash can also give useful clues in this context. Although the large normal variability of the amplitude of the occipital response to pattern reversal does not allow one to make as much use of amplitude information as one would like, the amplitude of the response from the two eyes in any one individual is usually very similar. In uniocular lesions, therefore, this information may be very useful. Uncorrected refractive errors will also affect the amplitude of the response, but, for a given acuity level, the reduction is much less marked than for retinopathy or axonal degeneration.

To summarise, the pattern evoked response has shown itself a very useful technique, particularly for the diagnosis of demyelinating lesions of the visual pathways. Delayed responses are not specific to multiple sclerosis; rather they seem to be associated with any demyelinating lesion of the visual fibres, and this may be produced by compressive lesions and some hereditary degenerations, such as Friedreich's ataxia, which are associated with segmental demyelination in the central nervous system. The method is as yet in its infancy, and a great deal still needs to be done to see how far its use can be extended, but it is already valuable enough to the practising neurologist and ophthalmologist to be included in the routine procedures in a go-ahead department of electrodiagnosis. It is, in fact, being introduced in a very large number of such departments all over the world at the present time.

References

Arden, G B, Bodis-Wollner, I, Halliday, A M, Jeffreys, A, Kulikowski, J J, Spekreijse, H and Regan, D. (1976) Methodology of patterned visual stimulation. In: Desmedt, J F (ed.) New Developments in Visual Evoked Potentials in the Human Brain. London: Oxford University Press. In Press.

Behrman, Joan, Halliday, A M and McDonald, W I. (1972) Visual evoked responses to flash and pattern in patients with retrobulbar neuritis. Electroenceph. clin. Neurophysiol. 33 : 445.

Cappin, J M and Nissim, Sarah. (1975) Visual evoked responses in the assessment of field defects in glaucoma. Arch. Ophthalmol. 93 : 9-18.

Dawson, G D. (1954) A summation technique for the detection of small evoked responses. Electroenceph. clin. Neurophysiol. 6 : 65-84.

Halliday, A M. (1968) Computing techniques in neurological diagnosis. Brit. med. Bull. 24 : 253-259.

Halliday, A M. (1972) Evoked responses in organic and functional sensory loss. In : Fessard, A and Lelord, G. (eds.) Activités evoquées et leur conditionnement chez l'homme normal et en pathologie mentale. Paris : Editions Inserm. 189-212.

Halliday, A M, McDonald, W I and Mushin, Joan. (1972) Delayed visual evoked response in optic neuritis. Lancet (i) : 982-985.

Halliday, A M, McDonald, W I and Mushin, Joan. (1973a) The visual evoked response in the diagnosis of multiple sclerosis. Brit. Med. J. (iv) : 661-664.

Halliday, A M, McDonald, W I and Mushin, Joan. (1973b) Delayed pattern-evoked responses in optic neuritis in relation to visual acuity. Transactions of the Ophthalmological Society of the UK. 93 : 315-324.

Halliday, A M, McDonald, W I and Mushin, Joan. (1974) Delayed visual evoked responses in progressive spastic paraplegia. Electroenceph. clin. Neurophysiol. 37 : 328.

Halliday, A M, McDonald, W I and Mushin, Joan. (1975) Abnormalities of the pattern evoked potential in compression of the anterior visual pathways. Australian Journal of Ophthalmology. In Press.

Halliday, A M, McDonald, W I and Mushin, Joan. (1976) Visual evoked potentials in patients with demyelinating disease. In: Desmedt, J F (ed.) New Developments in Visual Evoked Potentials in the Human Brain. London : Oxford University Press. In Press.

Halliday, A M and Michael, W F. (1970) Changes in pattern-evoked responses in man associated with the vertical and horizontal meridians of the visual field. J. Physiol. 208 : 499-513.

Halliday, A M and Michael, W F. (1972) Pattern-evoked potentials and the cortical representation of the visual field. In : Somjen, G G (ed.) Neurophysiology studied in Man. Amsterdam : Excerpta Medica. 250-259.

Halliday, A M and Pitman, J R. (1965) A digital computer averager for work on evoked responses. J. Physiol. (Lond.) 178 : 23-24P.

Hubel, D H and Wiesel, T N. (1962) Receptive fields, binocular interaction and functional architecture in the cat's visual cortex. J. Physiol. (Lond.) 160 : 106-154.

Hubel, D H and Wiesel, T N. (1968) Receptive fields and functional architecture of monkey striate cortex. J. Physiol. (Lond.) 195 : 215-243.

McAlpine, D, Lumsden, C E and Acheson, E D. (1972) Multiple Sclerosis: a Reappraisal. Edinburgh: Churchill Livingstone. 202pp.

McDonald, W I and Sears, T A. (1970) The effects of experimental demyelination on conduction in the central nervous system. Brain. 93 : 583-598.

Michael, W F and Halliday, A M. (1971) Differences between the occipital distribution of upper and lower field pattern-evoked responses in man. Brain Res. 32 : 311-324.

PERIPHERALLY EVOKED SPINAL CORD POTENTIALS IN NEUROLOGICAL

DIAGNOSIS

D. G. Small

University Department of Clinical Neurology

Churchill Hospital, Oxford, U. K.

Cerebral responses evoked by peripheral nerve stimulation and recorded from the scalp in man were first investigated by signal averaging over 20 years ago (Dawson 1954). Much has been learned of the normal response and of its alteration in disease but clinical applications have been limited. We have explored the possibility of recording from lower levels of the central sensory pathway and have reported a response which can be recorded over the back of the neck and base of the skull (Matthews, Beauchamp and Small 1974). It appears to be of nervous origin and is likely to be useful in the study of neurological disease, particularly in conditions such as multiple sclerosis where central conduction may be interrupted or delayed.

METHOD

The stimulus was a square-wave current pulse of 0.3 ms duration applied to the median nerve at the wrist. The recordings were made from chlorided silver disk electrodes applied to the skin over the cervical spinal cord and cerebral cortex. Routinely these were placed between the sixth and seventh cervical spines (C7) and immediately rostral to the second cervical spine (C2) with a common mid-frontal reference electrode (Fz, 10-20 system), and in addition the cortical response from the hand area of the contralateral parietal region was simultaneously recorded. The amplifiers had a flat frequency response from 2 to 1000 Hz and a high frequency roll-off of 24 db/octave above 1500 Hz. The signals were sampled digitally at 10 points/ms and averaged by summation of 256 responses.

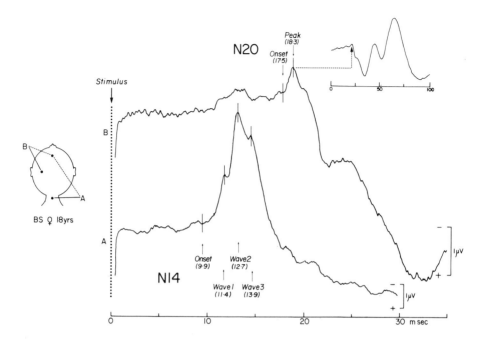

Fig.1 Cervical and cortical responses recorded simultaneously from an 18-year-old normal female, evoked by stimulation of right median nerve at wrist and averaged from 256 responses. Points at which measurements were made are identified on cervical (A) and cortical (B) traces. Small trace shows cortical response on slower timebase.

It was established in a preliminary investigation that with increasing stimulus current there was an initial steep rise in response amplitude accompanied by a moderate reduction in latency, both measurements levelling off at stimulus currents of approximately three times sensory threshold. In routine recordings, therefore, a current of four times sensory threshold was used, repeated at 1/s. This produced a tolerable twitch of the thenar muscles and was not painful.

NORMAL SUBJECTS

The cervical somatosensory evoked potential (SEP) in response to median nerve stimulation was examined in 30 normal subjects aged 18-53 years. A predominantly negative wave of complex shape

was recorded from all subjects (Fig.1, A). The mean amplitude
(onset to peak) was 3.0 μV (range 1.4-4.9). In different subjects
the onset and peak latencies ranged from 9.4 to 11.8 ms and from
11.9 to 14.3 ms respectively. Both these measurements were
strongly correlated with arm length (Fig.2). Comparison of the
cervical SEP with the cortical response recorded with a bipolar
montage (Fig.1) showed that the cervical response (N14) was
virtually complete before the onset of the first cortical
deflection (N20) at about 17 ms. Although there was individual
variation, three distinct peaks could be recognised within the
cervical SEP in all subjects. The major peak (wave 2) was

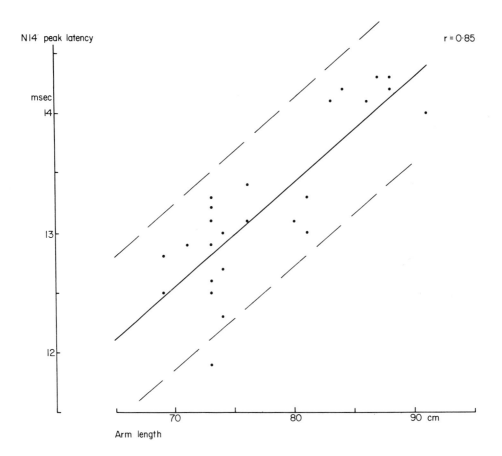

Fig.2 Relationship between peak latency of cervical response
evoked by median nerve stimulation at wrist and arm length
measured from wrist to seventh cervical spine (correlation
coefficient 0.85). Solid line is calculated linear regression
of latency on arm length and dashed lines are drawn two standard
deviations from mean.

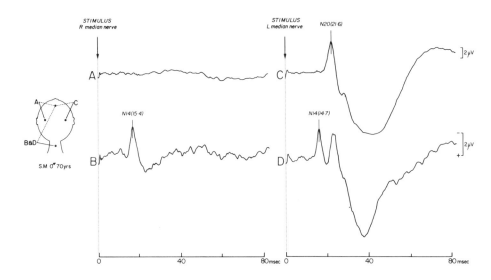

Fig.3 Cortical and cervical SEP recorded from a 70-year-old male following infarction of the left cerebral hemisphere. Cervical responses to both right (B) and left (D) median nerve stimulation are present, as is the cortical response to stimulation on the left (C), but there is no cortical response on the right (A). (Note slightly delayed cortical response appearing after N14 in D, arising from mid-frontal reference electrode).

preceded by about 1.3 ms by a minor peak (wave 1) and followed by a further minor peak (wave 3) after a similar interval. In all subjects in whom these peaks were clearly defined their latencies were identical when recorded at C7 and at C2. These observations have led us to suggest that the components of the cervical SEP may be generated from fixed sites within the CNS.

PATIENTS WITH NEUROLOGICAL DISEASE

In order to clarify the origin of the cervical SEP recordings have been made from patients with a variety of neurological disturbances (Small, Beauchamp and Matthews, in preparation). Preliminary results are reported here. Recordings from three patients with focal neurological lesions illustrate some of the major changes which have been found. The responses in Fig.3 were recorded from a 70-year-old man who had had a severe infarction of the left cerebral hemisphere. Stimulation of the right median nerve evoked no cortical response over that hemisphere, whereas there was a normal response over the healthy hemisphere to stimulation on the opposite side. In contrast, the cervical responses to stimulation on either side were normal.

The recordings in Fig.4 were obtained from a 41-year-old woman with a lesion of the brainstem and also show a dissociation between cortical and cervical response. Again normal cervical responses were found, while the cortical responses were clearly abnormal, being of low amplitude and having a delayed onset. The third illustrative record from this group (Fig.5) is from a patient with severe cervical myelopathy, secondary to spondylosis, and confirmed at operation. The cervical responses were absent and the cortical responses very small.

Data from such patients, where the approximate extent of the lesion is known, suggest that the scalp recorded SEP, beginning with N20, is generated in the cerebral cortex, and that the SEP recorded over the cervical region has a subcortical origin and is generated largely in the cervical cord.

We have also made recordings from patients with multiple sclerosis (MS), most of whom were in the very early stages of the disease. The recordings in Fig.6 were from such a patient who, at the time of examination, complained only of minor sensory symptoms in her right hand. Clinical examination revealed no objective signs of sensory loss. With stimulation of the left median nerve, both the cervical and the cortical responses were normal, but with stimulation on the right the expected cervical

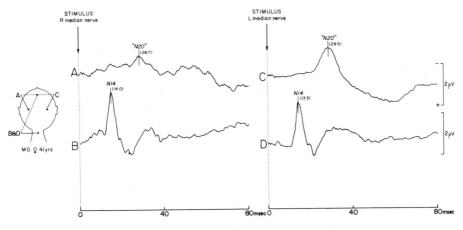

Fig.4 Cortical and cervical SEP from a 41-year-old female with an acute brainstem lesion. Cervical responses (B and D) are normal but cortical responses (A and C) are delayed, of low amplitude and of abnormal shape.

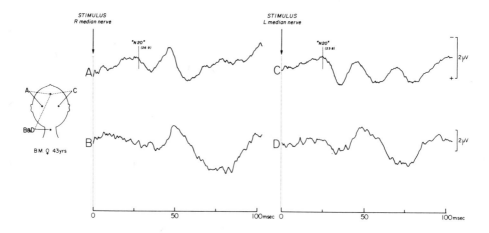

Fig.5 Cortical and cervical SEP from a 43-year-old female with cervical myelopathy. There are no discernible cervical responses (B and D) and the cortical responses are delayed and of low amplitude.

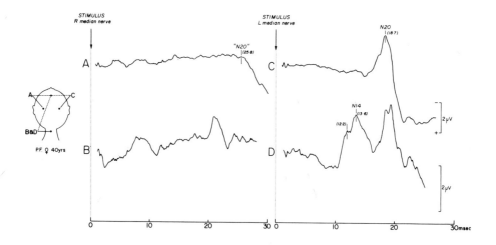

Fig.6 Cortical and cervical SEP from a 40-year-old female with MS. At the time of recording she complained only of paraesthesiae in the right hand, and clinical examination revealed no sensory loss. Cervical and cortical potentials from left wrist (D and C) are within normal limits. There is no cervical SEP from the right (B) and the cortical response (A) is delayed.

response was not present and the cortical response was of abnormal shape and delayed to nearly 26 ms (normal less than 22 ms). This patient thus had a unilateral neurophysiological abnormality on the same side as her subjective sensory symptoms with changes in both the cervical and cortical evoked response. The patient whose recordings are shown in Fig.7 had as her only complaint blurred vision in one eye, due to retrobulbar neuritis, and the remainder of the clinical examination was normal, but her subsequent clinical course was consistent with a diagnosis of MS. On the side illustrated, the cortical response appeared normal in shape and was not delayed, but there was no cervical response at the expected time. There was, therefore, neurophysiological evidence of an additional lesion before it had become apparent in any other way.

Another type of abnormality which was sometimes found is shown in Fig.8. These recordings are from a 34-year-old man who had had three episodes suggestive of demyelination in the past and at the time of examination a residual spastic paraparesis without sensory loss. Like the last patient, the cortical response was normal but the cervical response was of abnormal shape.

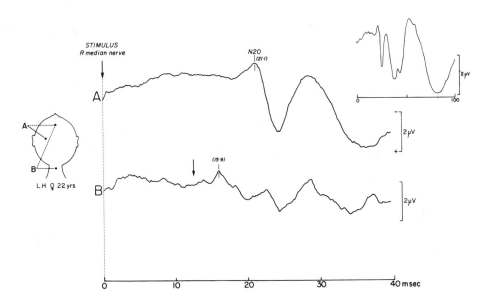

Fig.7 Cortical and cervical SEP from a 22-year-old female with retrobulbar neuritis, whose subsequent clinical course was consistent with a diagnosis of MS. There is no cervical response at the expected time, shown by the arrow in B, but the latency of N20 is within the normal range at 21 ms (A) and the shape of the cortical SEP (shown in small trace) is normal.

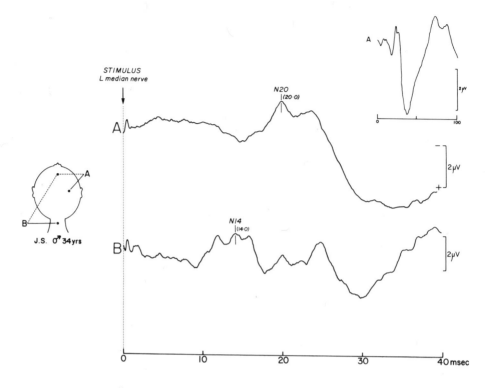

Fig.8 Cortical and cervical SEP from a 34-year-old male with spastic paraparesis due to MS, but without clinical signs of sensory loss. Cervical response (B) is of abnormal shape but cortical response (A) appears normal.

Over 100 patients with MS have now been studied. When the recordings of the cervical SEP from these patients were compared with those from the control group, differences in expected latency (predicted from arm length) and/or shape could be recognised in over 60 %. When the patient group was restricted to include only those with a "definite" likelihood of having the disease (McAlpine, Lumsden and Acheson 1972) or to those with clinical signs of abnormal function in the upper limbs, the abnormal proportion rose to nearly 90 %. These figures can be contrasted with an incidence of abnormality of the cortical SEP of 12 % and 47 % for the whole group and those with "definite" MS respectively.

The technique of recording the cervical SEP appears to be a sensitive method of assessing spinal cord function in MS and can provide information which cannot be obtained by other means.

Furthermore, in conjunction with recordings of responses to other modalities of stimulation (e.g. visual, auditory) it can suggest the presence of the multiple CNS lesions so characteristic of the disease. However, despite its possible diagnostic value in MS, a more important application of the technique may be as an objective method of studying the function of the cervical spinal cord in intact man.

This work was supported in part by the Multiple Sclerosis Society of Great Britain.

REFERENCES

Dawson, G. D. A summation technique for the detection of small evoked potentials. Electroenceph. clin. Neurophysiol., 1954, 6: 65-84.

McAlpine, D., Lumsden, C. E., and Acheson, E. D. Multiple Sclerosis: a Reappraisal. 202 pp (Churchill Livingstone, Edinburgh, 1972).

Matthews, W. B., Beauchamp, M. and Small D. G. Cervical somatosensory evoked responses in man. Nature, 1974, 252: 230-232.

PART IV

Clinical Measurements in Wards

GUEST LECTURE

Sir George Godber

Former Chief Medical Officer

Department of Health and Social Security

Madam Chairman, ladies and gentlemen, there are good reasons in the breadth of interest of your programme why I should be here to listen, but the only reason why I am a speaker - admittedly as a guest and amateur - is that Mr. Jackson Burrows has been my friend for many years and his genuine expertise has been exploited by me so many times that I could not refuse him now. Your programme is remarkable in range and content and I wish I were able to hear it all. It reads like a directory to the problems of science in medicine or medicine in science - I am not sure which way it should be put.

There will be time at the end of this talk for you to come back at me, so I will start by saying that your title is wrong. Why scientific aids to hospital diagnosis ? That implies that diagnosis outside hospital either owes little to science or it is involved with different science. Surely we don't think that; least of all this country where we have not only maintained and developed general practice but also come to a much clearer relationship between general and special practice.

Look at session one with its reference to screening. Where is screening likely to be important if not selectively in general practice with the immediate fall back position of reference to the relevant specialist if there is a positive finding ?

In session two the technicalities are highly specialised, but are we ready to use them yet for unselected populations and will we not rely on the family doctor for much of the communication with the patient, especially if there is to be follow up because of uncertainty?

Session three is perhaps a bit more esoteric but it still needs communication with the G.P.

Session four is specifically about the in - patient situation, though I guess there is a great deal of basic nursing done outside that situation and often by people who are not nurses at all. There are far more frail, old, even bed-ridden people at home than in hospital beds.

Session five is to be mainly about the hospital situation but I think it should contain something about the communication that has to be made to patients and relatives and as often as not by the G.P.

The G.P. does get a look in during session six, but it is about diagnosis.

I don't think your programme has given enough weight to that other great benifit of scientific measurement in medicine, the control of therapy and the precision it can give to prognosis. One of the things we must always remember is that the general public knows how much more precise medical science has become; it may be less intelligible in detail, but it is known or suspected in general terms and people expect to be told.

During the last few years all countries with sophisticated services have become increasingly pre - occupied with their cost. The main cause of the troubles of our NHS in the last two years has been the general shortage of funds. The money made available for the NHS has increased by only about one third while in Sweeden it has increased by about four fifths. Now we spend about one tenth of our national budget on health services, proper, or nearly one eighth if you include the related personal social services and we are only going to get more from higher taxation or by depriving some other service. Obviously we have to be sure that the money we are spending is necessarily spent.

Without the benefit of factual evidence or much thought a lot of people blame the wasteful use of scientific investigation, the drug bill or concentration on expensive activities like transplant surgery. Now all those things play some part, but I suspect we have taken far too little account of the increase in much more mundane activities like trying to do justice to the human needs of the patients in long stay care. The published returns show that between 1958/9 and 1972/3 the cost per patient week increased by 273% for acute hospitals, but by 337% for hospitals for the mentally ill and 335% for the mentally handicapped. I am not going to pursue this financial line further but have used it only to put the record straight.

There has been a great increase in the volume and variety of scientific investigation of patients and again it has not all been to serve the interests of hospital based doctors who do that; we must look carefully at the figures before drawing conclusions. In a twelve year period to 1971 the use of radiology as measured by values increased by 75%, but use by general practitioners increased by 131% to one ninth of the total. For Pathology the corresponding figures were a general increase of 158% with an increase of 429% for general practitioners to one seventh of the total. There have been plenty of reports from hospital departments to show that general practitioner use of diagnostic service is more, not less, discriminating than that by hospital staff.

In spite of these figures we must recognise some force in the allegation that too many investigations are done. I do not doubt that there are often also too few investigations. Medical audit is not a popular term here but it is still in much more vogue in North America where all too often it does describe a curiously mechanical review of medical care. The professional services Review Systems now being used seem to hark back to the old hospital acceditation system which had some of the same automatism. Nevertheless we do need to look a bit more qizzically at the use of investigative methods here. Automation has made it all too easy to accumulate paper information that is not always relevant to the state of the patient. Of course multiple chemical or other analyses do produce some unexpected and highly relevant information and we have not yet looked closely enough at the possible benefits of having in the patient's only continuous medical record - that held by the G.P. - a note of some of the parameters in a laboratory profile at different ages.

The finding might be just as relevant in adult life as the weight and height record during childhood or the weight during pregnancy.

I do not want to dwell on that, because there is a different point arising from automation in laboratories which is more relevant to your discussions. Automatic analysers of various kinds offer substantial savings in manpower for the work done, provided that it is not dissipated by doing too much work that is not needed. They also make standardisation of results in and between laboratories much easier. But these machines are very expensive if their range is wide, and they will only be acceptable as a cost of the service if they can be fully used. Like X ray plant they are at risk of early obsolescence, and they should be worn out rather than preserved. That means that we must expect to see some of the commoner work of laboratories concentrated. That in turn would mean concentration of pathology staff unless the role of the pathologist as an interpreter rather than a machine minder is accepted. Looking back over thirty years I can remember a lot of occasions when clinical specialists have behaved in a rather lordly fashion to those who do not spend so much of their time in direct contact with patients. I can also remember how thirty years ago some of the pioneers of clinical pathology like S.C. Dyke, Gladstone, Osborn and L.D. Thornton brought modern medicine to areas where the medical specialities developed only in their wake. It was sad to learn of the death of Dyke this year. He, Joseph Sheldon and Robert Milnes Walker together gave a new dimension to medicine in the Black Country. Sadly I have only heard the record half of this mornings session - just enough to wnet the appetite; even that was enough to point up one of the most urgent problems in the NHS today within the major problem which Mr Healey took $2\frac{1}{2}$ hours to instill into us all yesterday. We are going to be desperately short of resourses and even more restricted than a lot of other countries. It is going to hit us harder than they will be hit, because apart from Scotland, Britain has been under financed for the last 15 years at least. That has made us use what we had economically and left no margin at all. We must not use new techniques wastefully - things like Computer Assisted Tomography will not be cheap. But we must keep on supporting the leading edge and to do that we will have to develop selectively and economically. We cannot afford casual indulgence in new ploys. That is what makes a meeting such as this so important and the use of rational selection subsequently even more so.

Twenty four years ago at a group medical centre in New Jersey I saw radiotherapy equipment which was used only spasmosically by a diagnostic radiologist. I do not need to emphasise what a costly and even dangerous futility that was. We did not do such things in this country and we have to be even more careful now.

Medicine is less and less a single handed activity, despite the necessity of having one clinician firmly holding the ultimate responsibility in any episode. This point will presumably come out in the last contribution to session five. I believe that we have not yet developed the collaborative pattern far enough. We have for instance been singularly slow to develop the speciality of clinical physiology or clinical measurement or whatever we decide to call it. I believe we have one chair in the subject whereas Sweden had one in each of its medical schools nearly a decade ago. There is also still doubt in the minds of some doctors about the place of the non- medical scientist in the clinical field. I think that is going as it certainly should. There are chemists, physicists, engineers, micro - biologists and statisticians to name only some of the scientists in general hospitals and there are clinical psychologists who must surely play a much larger part in psychiatry in future. There are fields in which the management

of the social problems of an illness is at least as important as
the medical. We doctors have been getting the major part of the
blame for society's neglect of the mentally handicapped although
their problems are more social and educational than medical, and
doctors were among the first to experiment with the educational
approach, stimulated by the work of such as Jack Tizard and
Lionel Penrose.

I think we have a general problem in medicine that our concern
for continuing responsibility in the patient's interest has made us
too possessive both against intervention by other doctors and more
fiercely against people without the medical label. It is not
altogether suprising that in the middle of a defensive medical
debate about the propriety of giving social workers access to
medical records we suddenly become aware that the social workers
are at least as concerned about the fitness of doctors to have
access to their information. One gets the same reaction for the
same reason between phychologists and doctors. Now too one is
beginning to see an increasing reaction against the assumption by
doctors that they are always the leaders in the clinical context,
when sometimes nursing considerations should be paramount.

Just recently I came across a most interesting number of
"Search" the journal of the Australian and New Zealand Association
for the Advancement of Science. It was devoted to subjects
closely related to yours this week, but the paper most interesting
to me, written by Erica Bates, was about changes in the Medical
Profession. She discussed these inter - relationships much in the
terms I had already written for this afternoon. She made a most
important further point. There will not be an adjustment of
responsibility unless both the doctors are prepared to concede
and the other professions to accept responsibility: what we need
is not to transfer possession but to share. It is not a
possession anyway. Patients are their own people not ours.

The author of personal view in a recent issue of the British
Medical Journal, who is a Gynaecologist, makes this point from
his own personal experience far better than I can. I attended the
spring meeting of the Royal College of General Practitioners in
Dundee recently. During a very good symposium on evaluation just
this point was brought out. I was reminded once again that the
best General Practitioners are the guarantee of the humanity
which characterises British Medicine.

I suppose that in the present context I need to go on record as
believing that the NHS is not only going to survive but to progress,
and that there must be a workable settlement to the present dispute.
In spite of all the difficulties and shortcomings of the NHS we have
evolved a district unit which can give more an economical, more
continuous and ultimately more successful pattern of health care

than other systems with which I am familiar. Of course that pre-supposes that the money will be found. The large number of people now involved in providing comprehensive care requires proper exchange between them. This can be facilitated by various aids to communication which I am sure will include linked computer based records in the future. I think we must beware of thinking too much in such terms. The computer is a necessary mechanical aid, not a person. Communication is not fully effective unless it includes an element of personal contact. The most important place in any health distrcit in the future will not be the hospital. Primary care and preventive work are most important to the health of the people than the specialist care in hospital anyway. But that does not make the health centre the most important element either. Primary care is effective only if it can rely on the fallback position of the specialist help the hospital can provide. The postgraduate institute has become the focus of medical activity in almost every district in England and Wales - I omit Scotland only because I have not played any part in its development and do not know it. I look to the further progress of this postgraduate movement to keep British Medicine where it should be - in the forefront. The quality of medical care depends not on the latest scientific advance applicable to the treatment of just a few patients but on the way in which the ordinary jobs are done. That is not just a matter of scientific precision either; the appropriateness and humanity of what we do for patients is just as important.

Ivan Illich in his "Medical Nemesis " has maintained that the medical establishment, so far from being an asset, has become a threat to the health of the world. That book is worth reading for two reasons. First Illich is expressing in extravagant terms something which is at the back of the minds of quite a lot of people who have a faint suspicion that there are doctors to whom the patient is a walking lesion rather than a person, and who think in terms of the correction of a defect rather than helping a patient to the best functional result for himself. The two things are not always the same. That is why we get, periodically, accusations about experimentation on patients. We just cannot afford for ourselves or our profession to be anything but extremely careful on that point. The second reason why the book is worth reading is to observe how evidence can be misinterpreted and as a result, misused. Nevertheless there is enough in the book to make us uneasy and determined to make the allegations groundless in Britain. It is a fact that over 100,000 patients are admitted to hospitals in a year suffering from the adverse effects of drugs and it is unlikely that all those incidents were inevitable. Ten years ago there was that very unhappy episode of the excess deaths from asthma - several thousand of them - as a result of over-use of high pressure inhalants containing isoprenaline. Just before that there was the thalidomide tragedy. I do not mean that doctors could and should have avoided these incidents but they leave a natural uncertainty in the public mind that comes out at once on any hint of a risk with another drug. You will recall the backlash over heart transplants that many people believe reduced the chance of obtaining other donor organs, particulaly kidneys.

Communication within the profession is the solution to a lot of this. We have no place in the medical practice for secret remedies. But we have a long way to go before even the exchange of information between doctors working for the same patient can be regarded as adequate. I am sure I shall not be challenged here for saying that our medical records are in general not kept as well as they should be and are too often downright bad. They can be voluminous and detailed but still bad because they store information in an inaccessible way. Moreover the NHS sets out to provide continuity of care for a lifetime and the only linked record it provides is contained in a card and envelope used by the General Practitioner, usually of non-standard size and often padded out with hospital letters and test result forms of quite a different size and in random order. Eight years after the Tunbridge Report, hospital records are not even of a standard size. Here in the home of the Oxford Record Linkage Study there has been more progress than elsewhere, for which we should thank its founders Leslie Witts and Donald Acheson. A lot of General Practitioners egged on by their Royal College have advanced things themselves, but we have not made much use of the wonderful opportunity that the NHS should provide.

The King Edward Fund is currently interesting itself in improvement in this area and accommodated an interesting symposium on the problem Orientated Medical Record, organised by Dr. Neil McIntyre two months ago. It looks as if we really may be about to make some progress. We need to, because I believe that the worst failure of the NHS so far has been in the lack of review of clinical results. We are still preening ourselves on exercises like the confidential review of maternal deaths, or the perinatal mortality enquiry, when we should be asking about all the other comparable studies that should be made. There are some local activities and there have been many studies of clinical series, but not nearly enough systematic scrutiny of results. True the ORLS has done a lot here and we have HIPE but that is altogether too meagre a harvest.

It seems to me that it all comes back to our need to improve our methods of communication and our use of them. We must also be sure that we are not thinking just of medically qualified people. This session, I am glad to see, is about nursing, and matters of communication with patients on which nurses are better than Doctors - and need to be because they are the people in continuous contact with the patients in hospital at least. I have talked earlier about the part played by non - medical scientists , but there are all the nurses and the other professions that go to make up the Greater Medical profession proper. Fortunately there are signs that the rising generation of medical students has recognised this point and there are signs of grace in the postgraduate field. Last month I had the privilege of opening another multi-disciplinary postgraduate centre at a hospital - my fourth in two years.

Mr. Chairman I fear all this may have been rather off the beam, but I did not pretend it could be anything else. I really came here hoping to learn and expecting to do just that for the rest of the day.

NURSE - PATIENT - COMPUTER INTERACTION

Gillian Tobin

Clinical Teacher Intensive Therapy Unit

Westminster Hospital, London

The computer assisted charting and monitoring system was first introduced in May 1971. The system was designed and programmed at Westminster Hospital by the Medical Computer Department in conjunction with the medical and nursing staff.

As an aid to nursing care the system works by decreasing the time spent by the nursing staff, working in the cardio-thorasic Intensive Therapy Unit, in collecting, recording, and calculating fluid and colloid balances, temperature, venous pressure, blood pressure and pulse rate. This allows the nurses more time to spend observing and caring for the patient.

In the post operative period patients who have undergone open-heart surgery require vigilant, constant observation of cardiac, respiratory and renal function. This is achieved by recording blood pressure, pulse rate, central venous pressure, respiratory rate, tidal and minute volumes, urine output and blood loss, as well as crystalloid and colloid replacement. Prior to the use of the computer, the nursing staff made these observations, recordings and calculations every 15 minutes as well as carrying out routine nursing procedures for the patients.

FLUID BALANCE

Calculation of fluid balance was the first part of the computer programme introduced to the nursing staff. By using a hand held keyboard and the appropriate display on the Ferranti Visual Display Unit, nurses enter the fluid data. There are 14 codes under which crystalloid and colloid measurements can be entered.
To record an item of data the nurse types the code number, shown

on the left hand side of the screen, followed by a special function
key marked "reading" or "amount". Then the nurse enters the number
corresponding to the required data value followed by a further key
"EOF" which indicates the end of the entry. Immediately a message
confirming the entry is displayed in the top left hand corner of
the screen e.g urine amount 16 millilitres. This allows the nurses
to confirm the accuracy of her entry.(It is possible to cancel
the entry at this point or to correct it). Within 1 to 2 seconds
the item sub totals and overall balances are amended on the
display.

In the beginning both methods of charting were used
simultaneaously and this caused a great deal of work . The computer
always received all the blame for any discrepancies. Gradually
the nurses came to accept that provided they keyed in the correct
information then the balances produced by the computer would be
accurate.

Using this fluid data the computer produces various graphs
on the visual display unit in either 6 hour or 18 hour periods
of time.

        e.g. A. Crystalloid and colloid balance.

              B. Urine output and blood loss in half
                 hourly amounts.

Every 6 hours a typewriter automatically prints the fluid and
blood balance graphs which can be stored in the patients notes.
A complete record of each entry into the computer is kept in the
medical computer department.

PRESSURE RECORDINGS

Monitoring of cardiac function is achieved by means of cannulae
inserted into the right atrium, an artery and then connected
through transducers to the hewlett packard analogue boxes.
The electrocardiographic leads and rectal temparature probe are
also connected to theses analogue preprocessors.

A line selection unit which the nurses call "The Monitor Box"
was designed and made in the hospital. This allows IBM 1800
computer to sample data displayed on the analogue preprocessors.
This sampling takes place every 60 seconds. Every 5 minutes an
average of the previous 5 recordings is charted. The computer is
programmed to ignore any single value which differs greatly
from the rest when deciding which value to chart. All of these
values are constantly displayed on the visual display unit and
if the values are unacceptable a message flashes on
the screen "trace damping". There are switches on the

NURSE—PATIENT—COMPUTER INTERACTION

"Monitor Box" which enable the nurses to stop the sampling of incorrect data for which there are various causes, e.g. Artefact on the electrocardiographic trace will interfere with the accuracy of the pulse rate recording.

By using the appropriate display it is possible to enter these values using the keyboard.

Once these values are entered into the computer a visual display of the graphs is possible. These graphs are available in either 6 hour or 18 hour periods of time. Every 6 hours these graphs are automatically typed out. Although it is possible to key in the respiratory parameters this is not generally done because the values are not typed out on the charts.

FAIL SAFE

The fail safe measures were introduced in the autumn of 1972. They consist of a 30 minutely print out on the typewriter which gives all the current information about the patient, i.e. blood pressure, pulse rate, central venous pressure, rectal temparature, fluid balance, blood balance, and all the individual totals for the fluids. The typewriter is kept near but not in the ward because it is noisey and because there is no space. If it fails the computer is aware of the situation and has the charts printed by an alternative typewriter. If the paper jams in the typewriter this is not detected by the computer and it continues to have the 6 hourly graphs written on about $\frac{1}{2}$" of paper and the ward could be left without a written chart, therefore it is necessary to check the typewriter frequently.

STAFF TRAINING

Staff training still remains a problem. It takes longer to teach new members of staff to cope with the computer than to cope with the conventional charts. Once a new nurse has mastered the technique there is no doubt that:

        A/ She likes the new system.
        B/ She would always chose it in preference to any other method of charting.
        C/ It leaves her with much more time to nurse her patients.

SUMMARY

The computer assisted monitoring system began in May 1971 in the cardio thoracic intensive therapy unit.

The first stage was manual entry of fluid data which was

followed about 6 months later by automatic recording of pressures
The pressure recording was more easily accepted because the fluid
recording had convinced the nurses that the new system was efficient
Early 1972 it was possible to alter information about the patient
e.g. alter the urine output from 10 millilitres to 100 millilitres
2 hours previously. It was not untill all the fail safe measures
had been introduced that the conventional chart was discontinued.
Although it had not been used as an independant chart for some time,
it had been used just for recording the hourly fluid totals and
pressure recordings which had been copied from the visual display
unit.

THE PATIENT AND THE MACHINE

C.M. Roberts

Sister

Renal Unit, Royal Free Hospital, London

The human kidney has three main functions, the excretion of waste products of metabolism, the balance of salt and water in the body and the secretion of hormones associated with blood pressure control and the stimulation of the bone marrow.

In patients with chronic renal failure, one or all of these cease to function making it necessary to give some form of supportive therapy to maintain life. This can take the form of dialysis or renal transplantation. Dialysis is a substitution therapy by artificial means replacing the activity of the patient's own kidney. This only corrects the excretion of waste products of metabolism and the balance of salt and water, but obviously cannot correct the secretion of hormones.

Dialysis may necessitate the use of a machine by chronic renal failure patients to maintain life. Lay people often visualise the patient being placed inside a machine similar to an artificial lung, whereas medical personnel may think the patient lies prostrate connected to the machine keeping them alive. I wish to put in perspective the functions and use of the machine and its acceptance by the patient and their family.

There are two types of maintenance dialysis, Haemodialysis and Peritoneal Dialysis - both necessitating the use of a machine for unattended home treatment.

In haemodialysis, blood is taken out of the body, passed through an artificial kidney where osmosis and diffusion take place through a semi-permeable membrane and the purified blood returns to the patient. A proportioning machine mixes the dialysate, and pumps it through the artificial kidney, monitoring the temperature, flows and pressure continuously.

Peritoneal dialysis takes place inside the body using the peritoneum as a semi-permeable membrane as it has a large surface area, and is well supplied with blood vessels. Dialysate fluid is run into the peritoneal cavity where osmosis and diffusion take place and then the fluid containing waste products of metabolism is then drained by gravity and capillary action.

A simple automatic clamping device which enables unattended over-night peritoneal dialysis to take place was designed and made in our Renal Unit workshop. Two clamps are controlled by the timers above, which are set to the individual requirements. This machine is small and therefore portable and simple to operate.

In contrast, the haemodialysis kidney and machines are larger and far more complicated than the peritoneal clamping device and therefore the type of treatment chosen for each patient depends on their ability to cope, and the home situation.

Those patients on permanent home peritoneal dialysis are usually in the older age group who find it difficult to adapt themselves to new and complicated techniques. These patients range from 50 - 71 years of age. There are also a few younger patients with less intelligence who would find it impossible to learn haemodialysis techniques. By comparison, the haemodialysis patients range from 4 - 60 years old.

All forms of treatment are interchangeable according to the patients' needs. Home dialysis and transplantation are the only two forms of treatment that give the patient independence.

Adequate dialysis will maintain the level of blood urea and electrolytes within safe limits and the patients will feel fit and well during their treatment. But, if due to dietary indiscretions the patient expects the machine to do more than it is designed for, then he will begin to feel ill with headaches, vomiting or dizziness. It is these patients who do not adjust to dialysis and resent the machine.

In 1964 due to shortage of staff and lack of space in hospital, the first Home Dialysis was performed. Since then, all new patients are accepted for Home Dialysis be it haemodialysis or peritoneal dialysis. The Royal Free Hospital's first Home Dialysis patient used large metal tanks to store dialysate which are now replaced by smaller and safer equipment. This equipment changes rapidly with advancing technology. Also it is interesting to note the husband attended to the machine whereas now-a-days patients are taught to be independent.

Home Dialysis enables our 13 bedded Renal Unit to treat 139 patients, not including transplant patients, and the patients benefit with a high degree of rehabilitation and independence. Day and time of dialysis can be changed to fit the individual requirements, this is rarely possible in hospital with a fixed regime, thus the home patient spends more time with his family or persuing social activities and time is not wasted travelling to and from the Renal Unit which may be up to 200 miles away from his home.

When choosing equipment for Home Dialysis the following points must be considered. The most reliable equipment available is used. The machine must be automated with a short preparation time as patient's time is valuable. To give the patient confidence in the machine, it must have all reasonable safety devices. The patient must be able to move around whilst on dialysis and therefore independent. Although there are many disposable dialysers on the market, the cost and efficiency of these must be considered carefully. The equipment may be heavy and bulky and therefore the less it has to be moved the better, so the home must be arranged to accommodate it.

The siting and installation of the machine in the patient's home involves the patient, his family, the Hospital Home Dialysis Administrator and a building contractor. Where possible, a room separate from the bedroom is used for a haemodialysis treatment room. Care must be taken to look at the remainder of the family's needs as a whole, e.g. is grandma coming to live with the family, are there small children of different sexes who will in the near future need separate rooms? These are just a few points that must be taken into account. Unless the patient and family are happy with the idea of moving house, resulting in loss of support from friends and relatives, schools and employment, the policy of our Hospital is to find alternatives to rehousing. Adults usually dialyse at night and therefore a bedroom can be used. Children dialyse in the evenings and therefore ideally their treatment rooms are an extension of the living area where they are not isolated from the family, and mother can keep an eye on them whilst carrying out her household chores. For this, extensions may be built on to the home. Peritoneal dialysis, on the other hand, needs very little space and no adaptations. Some patients dialyse in the kitchen so they can continue with the cooking, washing up, etc.

TRAINING PATIENTS

Self Dialysis starts with the first dialysis. There is a regular day training school, five days a week, with a high staff to patient ratio during the day. Training is individualised and adapted according to the intelligence and comprehension of the patient. Varying levels of information are given to the patients, e.g. teaching the mechanics of the proportioning machine may result in a reliable helper who is able to fix technical faults alone, but on the other hand, the tinkerer may turn a minor fault into a major one. There is no formal training book and patients make their own notes. Patients are not fully trained on leaving the Unit but know how to communicate by telephone. Even children are taught the techniques of dialysis. When teaching the patients, the nurse must remember that a patient who is physically unwell may learn, forget and have to be retaught. Family participation is not essential but encouraged. During the patient's training period in hospital, the machine and treatment are gradually introduced to the patient's family. Particularly when the patient is a child, it is important to involve siblings. Children, family and friends can visit the patient whilst he is receiving treatment in hospital and the more gradual the introduction to the machine, the better the acceptance. Once the patient is competent to conduct his own treatment he commences dialysis at home. A Home Dialysis Sister remains with the patient for his first dialysis to give him confidence and relieve the family's anxiety. She will confirm his acquired knowledge of his treatment and gradually leave him alone to cope. She will revisit periodically - the frequency depending on the skill and confidence of patient and family. There is continued support for the Home Dialysis patient from the Renal Unit. A telephone is installed in all treatment rooms thus enabling the patient to call the Renal Unit at any time of the day or night for advice, whether it be medical, technical or a dialysis problem. There are always members of the Renal Unit staff available to deal with these problems.

It is hoped that the patient has found some member of the staff of the Renal Unit to whom he can relate his problems. Consideration at all times must be made for patients' commitments - whether they be at home or work and the patient should not be brought to the Renal Unit unnecessarily. To overcome boredom, regular holidays are encouraged - the patient may return for dialysis in the Renal Unit but alternatively may use the holiday dialysis kit designed by one of the Unit's doctors. Hospital dialysis is available for all emergencies. There must be an awareness of family's financial state. The Unit also provides a technical service for the machines. Any machine problems can be referred to the technician on call. Technical breakdown of the machine is not a matter of life or death as the patient's biochemistry is controlled so that dialysis can be delayed until the following day after repairs have been made. Major problems which are foremost for patients' concern are the withdrawal of supportive services over which the Unit has no control, such as Water Supply and Electricity. This can be remedied by communication by the services to the patient as to the date and time of cuts. If this is a long term problem, then a dialysis in the Renal Unit may be necessary.

All systems in the machine are monitored with numerous safety precautions making an audible and visual alarm to alert the patient - this cannot be overridden. In spite of this, one or two patients do not have complete faith in their machines and are concerned that a machine fault will occur and they will die whilst asleep. All equipment used must satisfy the Department of Health safety specifications - this produces complicated equipment and designers sometimes forget that the machine may be used by a person of limited intelligence.

Children sometimes see their mother as a manipulator of the machine and if problems arise they are related to the mother. Anxiety and frustration can arise from repeated minor technical faults which disrupt a family's planned programme. These faults become magnified as the machine then intrudes into the family and social commitments. To minimise these, technical equipment is serviced six monthly and interim problems are dealt with immediately by the Renal Unit technical staff.

Home patients anxiety relating to the machine can be overcome. This is not present in those patients dialysing in Hospital, but replaced by a greater anxiety which is more difficult to overcome - the competence or incompetence of the staff. Patients who have been dialysing in hospital for a long period of time may get very aggressive and suspicious of new staff and their ability.

Dialysis has changed considerably during the past 12 years. From one patient dialysing in hospital with four staff involved, we now have 117 patients at home alone with their machines with medical or technical help available on request.

To conclude, the dialysis machine must be viewed as a small essential part in a patient's treatment and must not be brought out of proportion. But its existence makes a full and active life possible for children and adults with Chronic Renal Failure.

KEEPING THE BALANCE BETWEEN BASIC AND TECHNICAL NURSING

AIDEEN PHILLIPS

NURSING OFFICER

WESTMINSTER HOSPITAL, DEAN RYLE STREET, LONDON S.W.1

To begin this talk I think it is necessary to give a brief outline of the circumstances that have led up to the situation as it is now, of keeping the balance between basic and technical nursing. With the advances of medical knowledge and treatment the nurse of today, though basically fulfilling the same role of caring for the patient, and carrying out treatment prescribed, has taken on a much wider field of work. Something that the nursing profession often asks itself is "Have Technical Advances Improved Patient Care". The answer to this must necessarily be yes, should be yes, and must, in the case of the nurse, be yes. Nurses as members of the major caring profession are concerned in the management of the total care of the patient, and therefore any means that are used to aid the nurse in this, must improve care.

Up to twenty five years ago the most complicated equipment most nurses had to deal with in the ward was various methods of drainage, the naso-gastric tube, tidal drainage, and underwater seal drainage. The output from these was measured and charted to be balanced against the input. Blood transfusions and intravenous fluids were given in very limited situations. Apart from this I think I am correct in saying that the only other clinical measurement done by the nurse was that of temperature, pulse and respiration. These were taken routinely twice daily or four hourly and charted, as they still are, and the importance of them has not changed. Perhaps the recording of a patient's respirations is now only done if it is abnormal, so that these are accurate, not showing every patient to have a respiratory rate of twenty per minute. The sphygmomanometer was used only by the doctor, and certainly the blood pressure was not recorded at frequent intervals as a means of observation, as we all accept today. When the nurse recorded the patient's pulse in the regular observation of the patient, she became an expert at assessing the condition of the patient by his appearance, his colour, the feel of his skin, just the way he looked. How important this still is, but perhaps with more advanced methods of measurement and assessment of patient's condition, do we continue to make the best use of our own senses, particularly those of sight and feel. Despite all modern technology, how often does an experienced nurse say "there is absolutely nothing to show it, but Mr So and So is not as he should be". She is nearly always right. I think we consider this to be our sixth sense.

Prior to the setting up of intensive care units in this country, machines were gradually being brought into use in the wards where they of course will still be used today. Twenty five years ago nurses working in fever and orthopaedic hospitals became familiar in the use of the "iron lung" and the Paul Bragg respirator for use with patients suffering from complete or partial respiratory paralysis following the severe epidemics of poliomyelitis in 1947 and 1949. In the late 1940's neuro-surgical units, some started during the war, as centres for the care of patients with head injuries, were expanding their work, and nurses working in this specialised field measured blood pressures as part of the routine care and observation of the patient. In the 1950's the use of intermittent positive pressure ventilation via an endotracheal tube was first developed in Scandinavia. Still in the 1950's cardio-pulmonary by-pass machines made possible more advanced cardiac surgery. These patients required post-operative monitoring of vital functions. So it continued into the 1960's, and new equipment which would affect the nurses' work was continually and rapidly being brought into use.

It was in the early part of the 1960's that it was seen that for the best use to be made of this equipment, for reasons of expense limiting supply, and especially that it may be used by people trained to use it, intensive care units were set up in this country, the first ones being found in side wards set aside for the care of patients following open heart surgery.

As today it is in these units that advanced technological nursing is carried out, I will give an outline of the role of the nurse in the Intensive Care Unit, her need to have specialist training to acquire the extra skills necessary to care for the patient, and to ensure the best use of technical advances by observation, interpretation and action, to maintain life during the acute phase of a patient's illness.

A Nursing Times editorial (1) in 1967 described intensive care nursing as "the zenith of technological nursing"; nurses in these units do work and care for the patient surrounded by mechanical and electronic machines, but his life depends not only on the machines but on the vigilance and capability of the nurse caring for him. There are many people alive today who perhaps would have died, but for the specialised care they received in an intensive care unit. Without this specialised care medical and nursing technology may work to the detriment rather than the benefit of the patient.

In the intensive care unit the nurse is seen primarily caring for the patient, carrying out basic nursing procedures so essential to both his physical and psychological needs. A patient during an acute phase of illness will probably be entirely dependent on those caring for him to carry out the normal functions of the body. His skin must be kept clean and dry, and free from any abrasions that may be caused by equipment or even a crease in the sheet. He must be turned frequently, usually two hourly, to relieve pressure, and even more important to aid drainage of any secretions from the lungs. Chest physiotherapy, and passive movements to all limbs, the latter to prevent further complications of contracture deformities which in turn slows down rehabilitation. Care of the eyes, nose and mouth; how distressing it is to see a patient where this has been neglected. The function of feeding preferably by the normal route of the stomach, if not contra-indicated, must be continued. This is usually via a naso-gastric tube, the diet containing the correct nutritional balance and calorie intake. There are still those that advocate that the dinner of meat and two veg, liquidised, cannot be beaten. Excretion of body waste must continue regularly.

Together with this basic practical care of the patient there is the important function of meeting the psychological needs of the patient. In the midst of all the equipment is a sick human being, often conscious, very anxious. His needs are those of an individual, a person. The nurse as well as meeting the needs of care and comfort, must at the same time use safely and effectively any equipment which contributes to the care of the patient. She must gain the confidence of the patient, so helping him to allow the machine to work to his advantage. She must be confident in her own ability to cope with any situation, this confidence being so important in reassuring the patient. Surely to be a patient dependent on a ventilator, to be faced with a nurse to care for you unfamiliar with the machine, must be a terrifying experience. The nurse has an important part in diminishing the effect of an anxiety producing environment. It is important that the nurse communicates with the patient by touch, by talking to him, many a patient can hear although unable to communicate. Every procedure must be explained to him. Discussion about the patient's condition or that of another patient must not be carried out by the bed. An ex-patient of an intensive care unit, himself a doctor, talking of his experiences to an audience of nurses, said that he could not understand why he had had a triple valve replacement performed and was not going to recover. It was days later that he realised it was the patient in the next bed that the doctors were discussing but moved from the patient's hearing, so causing great anxiety to another person. In meeting the psychological needs of the patient the nurse must include the emotional effect on visitors. When the patient most needs comfort and a link with the outside world he may be faced with a relative who sits looking terrified. The nurse must explain to the visitor, and encourage them to talk to the patient, hold his hand, reassure him. The nurse can learn a great deal about the patient in her care, from his relative. The need for care as an individual has been expressed in a book by an ex-patient of an intensive care unit in the words "In contrast to the cold steel of my respirator I wanted the touch of a warm human hand" (2).

You are probably thinking what has all this got to do with clinical measurements in wards, and keeping the balance between basic and technical nursing. I can only say a great deal. The nurse in the intensive care unit caring for a patient often surrounded and attached to machines by numerous leads and probes and tubes, must be aware and never forget the basic needs of the patient. In addition to this she must not only learn about the machine, but have an advanced knowledge of physiology and other sciences to understand the rationale of treatment, the changes which may take place in the patient and their implications for the nurse, and the effect on the patient as a social being. Only when she has enough of this knowledge and the skills to use it confidently can the nurse fulfil her function to nurse, in a technically advanced situation. She must be trained and efficient in the recording, and interpretation of all measurements. To do this she must be confident in her knowledge of the equipment in use. The nurse must be included from the very beginning in discussion on new techniques and the use of new mechanical aids. She must be able to advise from the nursing aspect, particularly, taking into consideration the effect this new procedure will have on her and the patient. If it detracts from patient care and takes the nurse away from the patient to use the machine, should she agree to this. Such technical advances will detract from patient care.

Results received for example, blood gas analysis, must convey to her that the patient is being adequately ventilated. She realises that the patient with hypo, or hyperkalaemia may have a sudden onset of cardiac dysrhythmia, she therefore observes this closely. The control of vital functions by use of drugs, the consequence of this action and appropriate regulation of the drug is within the nurse's work. A sudden change in fluid balance, diminished urinary output, the nurse must record, report and carry out prescribed treatment. These measurements are essential to the maintenance of life, but without the observation, interpretation and reporting by the nurse who understands their importance, much would be missed. However, the nurse is continually aware that as essential to life and eventual return to health the advances in technical aids are, what life will this patient have if he leaves hospital with a contracture deformity of his leg so confining him to a chair and further hospitalisation. Surely enough evidence of the importance of keeping the balance. In the early days of intensive care units a Consultant Anaesthetist, who admitted himself that up until his involvement in the unit he was removed from the ward situation apart from visiting patients, said to me "Sister, no matter how busy and chaotic the unit is, and whatever is going on, there is always a nurse somewhere combing the patient's hair, having just turned her, or changed her bed. I didn't realise that this was nursing and how important it is".

Nurses wishing to work in intensive care units today receive special training, most of them undertaking a recognised, though hospital based course, approved by the Joint Board of Clinical Nursing Studies. During this course they receive practical and theoretical teaching in all aspects of intensive care nursing, and at the same time further their basic skill as a nurse in the care of the acutely ill patient. To make such a patient feel and look comfortable is a skill, often made more difficult with technological advances. The cardiorator will tell us the patient's pulse but the nurse will still feel it and count it, during which time she is communicating with the patient. She meets his physical, emotional and psychological needs in the knowledge that the care of the patient has improved by advances in medical and nursing treatment and care. It has often been said and I regret still is said by many people "that nurses working in an intensive care unit are only interested in machines and not the patients". Someone trained as a technician, they omit to say which kind of technician, could do the work, it doesn't need nurses. I suggest to such people that they spend a day as an observer in a busy unit. It has been suggested that a trained intensive care nurse should be called a nurse technologist, I don't agree, she is trained as a nurse, a member of the caring profession who has acquired the expertise necessary to incorporate advances in medical treatment and technology in the care of her patient. She must always remember to, and keep the balance between basic and technical nursing.

References

1. Editorial 63.23
   The I.C.U. and The S.E.N.
   June 9, p 745, 1967 - Nursing Times

2. Carlsen R.
   The Unbroken Vigil
   Knox Press
   Nashville, Tennessee

PART V

Coordination and Communication of Results

CHAIRMAN'S INTRODUCTION

CHAIRMAN:

Barry Barber

Director of Operational Research

The London Hospital, Whitechapel, London. E1. 1BB

This morning's session is about information and communications systems. The word computer was deliberately left out of the session title in order that the emphasis should occur on the information and its use rather than on the computer technicalities. Computer systems have now been making headway in the Health Service for some fifteen years starting with routine finance and administration systems. This work has developed with sophisticated real-time computers handling the patient administration systems that deal with the broadly administrative information about patients that are the invariable preliminaries to medical care. Such systems have been linked with communications and service department systems and already one can begin to envisage the sorts of system that will handle patients' case notes. There are a number of severe stumbling blocks regarding the information to be included and the most convenient method of data capture. However, work is continuing at a number of centres throughout the world which must in due course lead to satisfactory systems. From there the way is open for computer assisted decision making systems which will give real help to the medical staff in carrying out their medical tasks as distinct from peripheral activities.
Such a development is indicated in fig. 1.

This morning's session looks to these more exciting development areas. Professor Alderson is concerned with the development of information systems within the re-organised Health Service suitable for monitoring the performance of the service in its provision of care and its use of resources. This material is basic to any rational Health Care planning, and it is relevant to the new D.H.S.S. Planning system. Indeed, the development of

FIG. 1.

DEVELOPMENT OF HEALTH SERVICE COMPUTING SYSTEMS

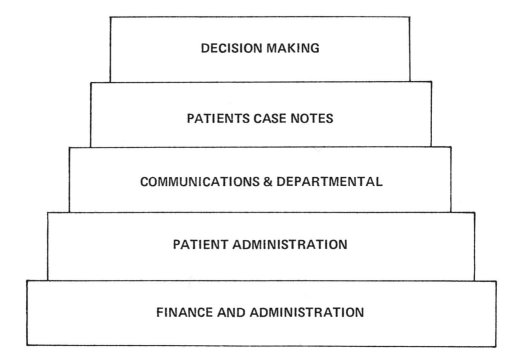

CHAIRMAN'S INTRODUCTION

really relevant information systems out of the present welter of poorly designed, poorly filled in and inaccurate forms supplied, reluctantly, to the Department of Health and Social Security is one of the challenges of the present time. Mr. de Dombal has for some years been concerned with computer aided decision making and he is well known for his pioneering work in testing pilot systems in specialist areas of medicine. It should be noted that such systems are of considerable value as aids to teaching as well as acting as a reservoir of the collective experience of the best way of handling particular problems. Dr. Clarke has been closely involved with medical computing at Manchester for many years and he will speak of some high level computer languages used specially for medical record data handling and analysis. Concluding the computer section, Mr. Abbott will speak of The London Hospital real-time computer system, its conception, birth and growth to date. He will also describe something of the effort required from senior hospital staff if such major systems are to be successfully implemented within such a complex multi-disciplinary environment as a modern acute hospital.

The last two papers from Mr. Steadman and Mr. Hambleton provide a glimpse of the power and versatility of present day microform systems. Such systems provide a very compact means of storing and retrieving information without the constant need for a large computer. However, microfilm and microfiche records may readily be generated from computer systems. The present limitations are that the devices for generating the microform output (COM) are generally fairly expensive to add to a computer system, although it is not expensive per 1000 pages reproduced or if one uses a computer bureau. Also, the facilities for entering data into a computer in microform fashion have unfortunately not yet become available. Mr. Hambleton's elegant use of basic diffraction physics to achieve multiple image storage on a single section of film considerably improves the packing factor of microform media for information storage - it also allows for colour reconstruction from black and white media.

This session should cover a number of matters that we may expect to hear more of in the future as the Health Service improves its information and communications systems to assist with the provision of appropriate, effective, and expeditious care for our patients.

REVIEW OF MEDICAL LINGUISTICS IN COMPUTING WITH SPECIAL REFERENCE
TO 'MUMPS'

D. E. Clark, T. C. Sharpe, A. J. Duxbury

University of Manchester, Medical Computing Unit

Coupland Building No.1, Manchester M13 9PL

Computers were first used in medicine in the U.K. in 1953. The first computer at the National Institutes of Health in Washington was delivered in 1958. Computers have until recently been difficult to use for processing medical data. In the early sixties the American Government invested a considerable amount of money in computers in medicine, and some of this was spent at the Massachusetts General Hospital (MGH) where attempts were made to computerise the hospital. Bolt, Baronach and Newman, the consultants in this venture, used a modified version of the interactive computer language 'JOSS' which ran on a PDP-1 computer sited remotely from the hospital. On this machine the language was called 'TELECOMP' but refined for medical purposes it became 'MEDCOMP'. A great deal of work was done in the hospital but progress was slow and difficult, and the need for a simple high-level language for medical work was evident.

Other workers had developed languages for handling medical record data. The free text system was developed by Korein[1] at New York University. The variable field, variable format system was developed by Sweeney[2] and Co. at Tulane, and on the West Coast Lamson in association with IBM[3] developed QPL, written in PL1. The other two languages were written in machine code.

The need for on-line working was evident, but should the language be an in-core compiler, or an interpreter? The compiler occupied about 4 times the core of an interpreter system but it is two orders faster. The other alternative is a phased system where compilation is only half the process, the rest being done by the loader or link editor.

Workers in medical data processing e.g. Pratt[4] at NIH, Wingert[5] in Munster, and Sharpe and Clark[6] in Manchester, have tended to favour the last view for practical working.

Medicine has 3 basic requirements, they are Service, Education, and Research, and Service brings the need for Service Packages. There is the need to be able to quickly adapt languages so there has to be a compromise between the speed of action and the ease of use. The main requirements for the language are:-

1. Automatic file handling and control of data, with infinite length for local and global arrays.
2. Text handling features as in 'SNOBOL'[7] and 'COMIT'[8].
3. Limited numerical features - minus, plus, multiply, divide, integer.
4. Line by line working.
5. Ability to address slow ADC's (1,000 samples/sec maximum).
6. Simple to use.

Extensions of 'BASIC' have most of the above features, but the language was not available for small machines in the mid-sixties, though the interactive language 'FOCAL' was available for the Digital Equipment Corporation of Boston (the makers of the PDP-1).

Any language had to be semi real-time and would have to work on small machines. Since it was evident that the development of a Hospital Interactive System was going to be difficult, the American Government withdrew support for larger machines to support the medium/small machines. At the MGH this meant DEC's PDP-9 and PDP-15. These machines could have multiplexors for VDU's and T/T's added to them. The language 'FOCAL' appears to have helped Dr. Roger Greenes and Neil Papillardo (the inventor of MUMPS) to develop a language that was powerful in its text manipulation features. The advantage of such a language soon became clear to workers in the field.

How MUMPS Works

'MUMPS', or the Massachusetts Utility Medical Program System is an interpreter. The interpreter reads in the user program, stored as source code, and adjusts itself to deal with the user data as dictated by the user program. Each pass of the user program means a full translating interpretation of the variables, so in practice this means that the system runs 150 to 300 times as slow as a compiled program. An example that we tested used 4 seconds of CPU in Fortran, but when run through a BASIC interpreter took 168 seconds.

In the 'MUMPS' system there is a time sharing/monitor and the machine normally allocates 50 milli-second time slices to each user. A user should ideally get a one second or less response in order not to slow down this thinking. However, this is not the data rate achieved, for instance the mean time between key depression on the Massachusetts Institute of Technology project MAC system was about 30 seconds.

The system occupies about 4k of core on a PDP-9, and users get allocated 4k blocks. If the user program is long, then it is swapped in and out in 4k blocks (which is approximately the amount of data on one disc swap).

Up to 15 users' with T/T's, VDU's and light pens, can use the system at any one time on a 64k memory machine. The backing Input/Output device on which the system depends is fixed and/or moving head disc, 3mch or 40mchrs. If the disc usage is low the user will get a time slice of 50m/s and the next user is activated, and so on. Each user is guaranteed a slice of time. The cost of these mini-computer systems varies from £275,000 down to £20,000$_{10}$.

Generally it is claimed that response time is 0.5 seconds per user; observing this unrelated system working of different problems the response times were as follows:-

a) Large program working with only 6 other users active - 24 secs. 5.15p.m.
b) Large data search with 2 users active - 24 to 30 secs. 3.15p.m.

A system may have a special disc tidying-up routine which is brought into action half-hourly to dump unused data onto magnetic tape. Larger user programs are automatically segmented and put out onto disc. An example is the Acid-base program which runs to some 50 pages.

Machine Environment

The language has the following instructions similar to FOCAL:-

BREAK	- provides an access point within the standard for non-standard programming aids without arguments, suspends execution until receipt of a signal, not specified here.
DO	is a generalised subroutine call.
ELSE	- sets a condition to be met.
FOR	- specifies repeated execution as the specified parameters.
GOTO	- is a generalised transfer of control.
HALT	- cause termination of the execution of this routine.

IF	- logical test
KILL	- sets specified variable to zero.
QUIT	- unconditional end of routine.
READ	-
SET	- assigns values to variables.
VIEW	- examine machine-dependant information.
WRITE	-

Functions

$ASCII	- selects a character of a string and returns its code as an integer.
$Z	- reserved for definition of implementation - specific function.
$CHAR	- translates a set of integers into a string of characters whose codes are those integers.
$DATA	- returns an integer specifying whether a defined value and/or pointer of a named variable exists.
$EXTRACT	- returns a character or sub-string of a string expression, selected by position number.
$FIND	- returns specifying the end position of a specified sub-string within a string.
$LENGTH	- returns the lowest numeric subscript value on the same level, but numerically higher than the last subscript of the named global or local variable.
$PIECE	- returns a string between two specified occurrences of a specified sub-string within a specified string.
$RANDOM	- return a pseudo-random number in a specified interval.
$VIEW	- reserved for implementation - specific methods of obtaining machine dependant data.

Special Variables

$HOROLOG	- provides date and time in a single two-part value.
$IO	- identifies the currently assigned I/O device.
$STORAGE	- provides the number of characters which are available in a routines partition.
$TEST	- makes available the truth value determined by the IF command and by the ASSIGN & READ with time outs.
$X	- gives the horizontal cursor position on the current device.
$Y	- gives the line number on the current device.

The language has the ability to time out a variable, i.e. if the data requested does not appear in a given time then the program can take alternative action, this is a unique R/T ability. The arithmetic is in 64 integers i.e. positive or negative 32 bit variables. The maximum instruction rate appears to be 5,000 to

10,000 user program instructions per second. This means that the line or statement rate is between 1,000 and 5,000 per second. Guessed at, the maximum processor rate for ADC is about 4k (single use). On a multi-user system this goes down to 4 samples per second, which is suitable for chemical pathology on-line and single user ECG systems.

Areas Where MUMPS is Used in Medicine

There are currently a host of about 200 medical user installations in N. America, most of them being in the U.S.A. The National Bureau of Standards is standardising the language, but currently there are some 10 versions available. Interest and use of the system has been expressed in Holland, France, Germany, Belgium, Denmark, New Zealand, Israel and England. The system is used in a) Patient Administration, b) Medical Data, c) Education, d) Research. In Patient Administration, since the language is designed to process text, it is easy to develop patient care plans; the Beth Israel Hospital has some 6 programmers working on this. In the areas of Medical Data Processing, Education and Research the MGH has a staff of 30 programmers and there are 5 computers on-line and active in the hospital.

Typical medical areas which include teaching, written by MGH and other hospitals are:-

a) Acute Respiratory Care.
b) Acid-Base Balance.
c) Chemical Pathology Reporting System.
d) Medical History.
e) Pulmonary Function.
f) Radiation Therapy.
g) Clinic Scheduling.
h) Clinical Data Analysis System.
i) Automated History Driver Programs.
j) Education:-

    1. Care of the unconscious patient.
    2. G.I. Bleed.
    3. Paediatric Problems, Cough, Fever, Jaundice.
    4. Abdominal Pains.
    5. Acute Cardiac Failure.
    6. Diabetic Ketosis.
    7. Cardiac Simulation.
    8. Examinations a) 36 signs, b) 33 disease conditions.

k) Nursing Notes.

64% of users of the system are medical school/university complexes.

A simple program which accepts results entered by a laboratory technician and stores them into this structure is shown below:-

```
1.10   READ !,"PATIENT ID   ",ID IF ID="" QUIT
1.15   IF 'ID:3N"-"2N TYPE "ILLEGAL ID FORMAT" GO TO 1.1
1.20   SET IDA=$PIECE(ID-1),IDB=$PIECE(ID-2)
1.30   SET ID = $VALUE(IDA)+$VALUE(IDB)/100
1.40   READ !,"TEST NAME",TN
1.50   SET TNN=$BOOLEAN(TN="NA",1;TN="K",2;TN="CL",3;TN="BUN",
       4;1,0)
1.60   IF TNN=0 TYPE " TEST NOT IN DIRECTORY "GO TO 1.4
1.70   READ !,"RESULT",RST
1.80   SET D=$DATE,DA=$EXTRACT(D3,4),DB=$EXTRACT(D,1,2)
1.85   SET DAR=$VALUE(DA)+$VALUE(DB)/100
1.90   OPEN ↑Z SET ↑Z (ID,DAT, TNN)=TN",".RST CLOSE
```

Comments for the above program:-

1.10   GET PATIENT ID NUMBER; IF NONE, QUIT
1.15   ASSUME ID IS OF FORM XYZ-NM. CHECK ID NUMBER FOR CORRECT FORM
1.20   BREAK ID UP INTO IDA=XYZ AND IDB=NM
1.30   SET ID (WHICH WAS A STRING) TO THE NUMBER XYZ.NM.
1.40   GET THE TEST NAME
1.50   CHECK THE SIMPLE DIRECTORY
1.60   IF NOT IN DIRECTORY, INFORM TECHNICIAN AND LOOP BACK TO 1.40
1.70   GET THE RESULT
1.80   AND 1.85 TAKE DATE, $D, WHICH IS IN THE DDMMYY AND BREAK IT APART INTO DA=MM AND DB=DD. THEN FORM DAT=MM.DD
1.90   ENTER THE RESULT INTO THE ARRAY ↑Z. THE OPEN ↑Z .. CLOSE SEQUENCE INSURES THAT NO OTHER TERMINAL WILL BE SENDING VALUES INTO ARRAY ↑Z WHILE THIS RESULT IS BEING ENTERED.

Advantages and Disadvantages

a) Advantages

1. System is very easy to use, and has powerful string processing facilities.
2. Program development, line by line for syntax checking is very good for the novice programmer, and also changing

programs is very quick and easy with the editing facilities.
3. The system will run on 12 or 16 bit machines, and will work on DEC's range, Data General machines, and special machines designed for the system.
4. Can take up to 15 users simultaneously.
5. Many packages have been written and there is a users group (MUG).
6. The system bridges the gap between medical administration (e.g. clinic scheduling) and medical data handling.

B) Disadvantages

a) Poor arithmetic, only integer working.
b) System occupies the whole machine since it is R/T.
c) Disc queue develops for programs and data.
d) Utility needed to clear disc half hourly, and for continuous high usage interactive load there is a need for very careful system programming.
e) Interpreter runs at 150th to 300th speed of compiled program, therefore the machine quickly becomes saturated.
f) It is unlikely to ever have a compiler version working as it stands.

Other Approaches to Text Processing

The European and American work mentioned previously shows that a very high volume of medical data and data retrieval techniques must run as fast as possible, this means that the source program must be compiled. High-volume of data means that the data must be passed into and out of core in an overlapped fashion, calling for a different machine structure using 32 to 36 bit words.

Complex text processing algorithms are being developed, e.g. the SNOP based system of Dr. Pratt and the segmentation algorithm of Wingert using extended SNOP and SNOMED. Sharpe and Clark are extending the segmentation algorithm using and adding Macro-search instructions. Once this work is done the system for processing medical text can be run on small machines if interactive usage can be kept low, 5 users per machine. Our own work is written in Fortran $\underline{IV}$. It will interface with the MUMPS$_2$ data bases through the CONFORM[11] system on input, and with SPSS[12], BMD[13], and other Fortran Data Bases on the output. Some simple machine code routines would make our output useable by the MUMPS system. We have gone to great length to make sure that text processing, statistics, number crunching and signal analysis are runable using a standard language such as Fortran $\underline{IV}$. The above mentioned searches are in binary and run at full speed on multi-overlapped channels, this is necessary due to the sheer volume encountered by the system.

MUMPS Development

There is now an American Bureau of Standards Committee whose purpose it is to define and standardise the MUMPS language. The interim language specification and transition diagrams have been agreed and defined. Associated with this Committee is the MUG (MUMPS User Group), and the MDC (MUMPS Development Committee), set up to facilitate the exchange of medical packages.

We can expect to see manufacturers other than the Digital Equipment Corporation and Data General with MUMPS interpreters.

In order to facilitate the use of packages developed, the NIH has sponsored a version of MUMPS written is Fortran $\underline{IV}$, and a 360/370 machine code version written by Jerry Wilcox[14] at Davis.

We $\underline{are}$ developing an English version of the MUMPS program in Fortran $\underline{IV}$ with a few machine code routines. The syntax checker is working. Hopefully, it can then be made to run on most university and polytechnic machines.

Summary

MUMPS as a language arose out of the need to be able to develop medical programs on smaller computers. Written as an interpreter it is easy to use and has very powerful text processing facilities. It has the advantages of being able to be completely self contained and run up to 15 users interactively. The major problem with the language for medical work is the large amount of disc activity whereby disc is used as back-up store. This results in a problem of slow response times with large data throughputs. Against this is the language is now in a standard form with many medical packages written for it. The arithmetic ability of the system is limited and number crunching problems are best tackled with the standard Fortran/Algol languages. As a result of ease of use and access the system is useful for medical data collection and for developing medical teaching programs.

Since MUMPS was first developed many small and medium size machines have acquired interactive facilities. The BASIC language is available in interpreter and compiler form.

In general, medical staff pick up programming languages after 2 or 3 hours tuition on an interactive terminal.

The language certainly speeds up the development of a program, but large volumes of data and large programs as a result of all the logic error checking which must go on, causes a queue for the disc on the small single highway machines.

The system may improve dramatically if all completely developed modules are put into machine code, and run in a 'round robin' time-slicing technique. We feel the language has the potential for medical work, and are implementing our own portable version.

References

1. Korein et al. Computer Processing of Medical Data by Variable Field Length Format. JAMA, June 1966, vol. 196, No.11.
2. Sweeney et al. Tulane Information Processing System. Tulane University Computer Science Series, 1965.
3. Cantor, D., Dimsdale, B., Hurwitz, A. Query Language One. IBM Form No. 320-2627, June, 1969.
4. Pratt, A.W., Automatic Processing of Pathology Data. Leaflet published by National Institutes of Health, Bethesda, Maryland.
5. Wingert, F. Word Segmentation and Morpheme Dictionary for Pathology Data Processing. Proceedings of the Medinfo '74 Conference, Stockholm, August, 1974.
6. Clark, D.E., Sharpe, T.C., Yates, P.O. 'MUMAS'. Proceedings of the Medinfo '74 Conference, Stockholm, August, 1974.
7. Desautels, E.J., Smith, D.K., An Introduction to the String Manipulation Language SNOBOL. Programming Systems & Languages, by Saul Rosen, published McGraw-Hill. pp 419.
8. Yngve, V.H., COMIT as an IR Language, Programming Systems & Languages, by Saul Rosen, published McGraw-Hill. pp 375.
9. Scherr, A.L. An Analysis of Time-Shared Computer Systems. published M.I.T. Press, Cambridge, Mass.
10. Glueck, B.C. Use of a Psychiatric Patient Record System. FASEB Federation Proceedings, December, 1974, vol. 33, No.12.
11. Sharpe, T.C. Analysis of Free-Text Medical Records by Computer Programs Written in a High-level Language. M.Sc. Thesis, University of Manchester Institute of Science & Technology, 1973. pp 56.
12. Nie, N.H., Bent, D.H., Hull, C.H. SPSS. Published McGraw-Hill.
13. Dixon, W.J. BMD. University of California Publications, Berkeley.
14. Wilcox, J. Personal communication. Details of an N.I.H. contract.

PROGRESS TOWARDS HEALTH INFORMATION SYSTEMS

Michael Alderson

Professor of Medical Information

University of Southampton

A health information system has been defined as "a mechanism for the collection, processing, analysis, and transmission of information required for organizing and operating health services, and also for research and training" (Alderson, 1973). This definition, terse as it is, implies that there are four rather distinct aims of a system - to assist management, to aid clinical study, to facilitate research, and to serve as a tool in teaching. During this talk I shall be concentrating on the first aim. In order to put the topic in perspective it is worth recalling that Florence Nightingale (1863) advocated the regular collection of a wide range of standard particulars to ascertain the results of particular treatments and special operations. She also suggested that the whole question of hospital economics as influenced by diets, medicines, and comforts could be brought under examination and discussion. Florence Nightingale was also keen to extend the study of data to out-patients. I will endeavour to distinguish ideas such as those of the 19th century pioneers from current practice and plans for the future.

One of the main functions of an information system is to monitor the performance of the health service; this can be considered at three rather different levels: - monitoring the public health at national level, reviewing the use of resources at district level, and auditing the outcome of care at individual level (patients or doctors). It has been suggested that the aims of the health service are to provide an available and acceptable service that identifies curable disease and makes the best possible use of resources. I shall now provide a few examples which indicate how routine data has been used to check upon these issues.

One aspect of the functioning of the services is of course measures of 'delay'; an example of this is the statistics that are prepared on the average waiting time to admission for patients who have been on a waiting list; this material is published annually by diagnosis together with aggregate counts of the total size of the waiting list by specialty in each district in the country. A rather different aspect of availability of the service is a range of analyses that are possible on the demand for and provision of services across the country. The annual reports on abortion enable one to look at the percentage of women having an abortion who go outside their region of residence to have this performed (OPCS, 1974). This varied from about 11% to 60% in 1973; this extreme range cannot be accounted for by variation in the wishes of the women to have this procedure performed elsewhere, but must in part reflect major variation in the availability of local facilities. Even if health service facilities are available it is important to check whether they are systematically used; a number of studies suggest that those in greatest need may in fact make least use of the facilities. For example, data from the perinatal mortality survey showed that those mothers with the highest perinatal mortality rate made the least demands upon specialist services, whilst mothers in social class 1 and 2 made the greatest use of the facilities (Butler and Bonham, 1963). Without wishing to enter the confusing field of the assessment of the value of screening, I will just mention that special surveys have been done on sub-groups of the population, which have identified conditions for which subsequent medical intervention has resulted in relief of symptoms. In particular surveys of the elderly have demonstrated a relatively high proportion of patients suffering from a whole range of physical and social handicaps which can be alleviated (Andrews et al, 1971).

A number of years ago Heasman (1964) used the 10% sample data from hospital discharges to look at the variation in length of stay for specific categories of patients. He showed that the average length of stay for patients having a repair of an inguinal hernia in different hospitals in the country varied from three days to twenty days (I must emphasise that this was the average stay for all such patients in the hospital and not just the scatter of stay for individual patients). It must not be thought that the simple examination of such material immediately enables one to comment on what is the correct use of such issues by a number of special studies. Where randomised controlled trials could be carried out there is a likelihood that definitive answers may be approached. This is still not an absolute occurrence as demonstrated by a study on the 28-day mortality of men with acute myocardial infarction who were treated at home or in intensive care units in hospital (Mather et al, 1971). Random allocation was only possible in a proportion of the patients; however, both amongst those randomly and electively treated at home there was a lower mortality compared with the hospital treated patients. This study is being followed up by further work but prompts me to emphasise the need to consider use of resources and outcome before making any judgement about alteration of the organisation of medical care.

Routine data facilitates relatively crude examination of outcome of care; I have arbitrarily selected two sets of data which may be used in this way. Examination of the death rate of children from measles and diphtheria over the past 100 years enables some comments to be made about the resolution of what was once an extremely severe medical problem - though the part played by preventive inoculation is not absolutely clear cut. Routine hospital discharge data enable case fatality to be examined in relation to characteristics of the patient and of the treatment. For example Heasman and Carstairs (1973) have demonstrated variation in the case fatality for patients treated for hyperplasia of the prostate.

I have spent some while discussing the range of uses to which information is presently put. I shall now turn to more specific comments about the present state of information systems and the rate at which they are evolving. Since the advent of the health service the DHSS has been supporting the gradual development of a range of statistical series, often in conjunction with the OPCS. The most detailed system relates to patients who have had a spell of inpatient care. There are existing systems for patients discharged following care in acute hospitals and for admissions to and discharges from psychiatric hospitals; an extending pilot of collection of data for maternity patients is in progress. Each of these systems collects brief particulars about the characteristics of the individual patient, the administrative arrangements for their care, and limited medical data. If arrangements are made to link subsequent admissions the range of analyses possible is greatly extended; the information is converted from event data to extending files of information about people. This enables more detailed examination of the patterns of care and of the outcome of care. The present systems only record limited particulars about use of theatres; only when data becomes available on nursing dependency, use of drugs, laboratory investigations, and x-rays will a more realistic picture be obtained of the use of resources for inpatient care. Over the past few years there has been a growing tendency to introduce day-surgery, or in other fields the use of day-hospitals; these complement the traditional care from outpatients and hospital wards. Only by the extension of the system to cover these aspects of hospital care will the aims mentioned in the earlier part of the talk be approached.

Though the hospital service is the expensive segment, the bulk of patient contact occurs in the community and the family doctor plays an important part in determining the use made of direct access investigation and the complete range of hospital facilities, in addition to the uptake of community services. Two national morbidity surveys have collected particulars about patient contact in primary medical care, but these have involved less than 1% of the population and are far removed from the development of routine sampling surveys of this aspect of the health service. Recently the General Household Survey has been established and will provide most useful information about the health of the population and the degree of self-care and self-medication. Many of the documents on the reorganisation of the health service have stressed the importance of assessing the health care needs of the population; measures of workload and outcome are dubious indices of need. Until the health information system covers need/demand/workload/use of facilities/outcome, management and planning in the health service will have to rely on judicious interpretation of routine data, the mounting of special surveys for major issues, and the use of modelling to fill the gaps in available data. Whichever approach is selected there will always be the over-riding need for judgement.

REFERENCES

Alderson, M.R. (1973). Objectives and concepts of Health Information Systems, EURO 4914/6. Working Paper prepared for Regional Office for Europe Conference on Health Information Systems, Copenhagen 18-22 June 1973.

Andrews, G.R., Cowan, N.R., and Anderson, W.F. (1971). The practice of geriatric medicine in the community. In Problems and progress in medical care, 5th series, ed. McLachlan, G. Oxford University Press, London.

Butler, N.R., and Bonham, D.G. (1963). Perinatal mortality. Livingstone, Edinburgh.

Heasman, M.A. (1964). Lancet, $\underline{2}$, 539.

Heasman, M.A., and Carstairs, V. (1973). Quoted by Doll, R. (1973). Proc. roy. Soc. Med., $\underline{66}$, 729.

Mather, H.G. et al. (1971). Brit. med. J., $\underline{3}$, 334.

Nightingale, F. (1863). Notes on hospitals, 3rd edition. Longman, Green, London.

Office of Population Censuses and Surveys (1974). The Registrar General's Statistical Review of England and Wales for the year 1973, supplement on abortion. HMSO, London.

PROGRESS TOWARDS COMPUTER-AIDED MEDICAL DECISION-MAKING

F.T. de Dombal

Reader in Clinical Information Science

University Dept. of Surgery, General Infirmary, Leeds

In talking about the use of computers in medical decision making, it is necessary to start from a point of considerable scepticism. For up to the present time, very few computer-aided systems have provided anything of value. Perhaps one of the main reasons why this is so is a question of semantics; and the fact that the two disciplines, computer science and medicine, are fundamentally different. In Leeds during the last four years we have investigated computer-aided diagnosis and decision making and it may be relevant to outline our experience, as an indication of the sort of potential benefit and practical problems associated with computer-aided decision-making.

FUNDAMENTAL CONCEPTS

Before dealing with the details of any one system, it may be helpful to discuss some fundamental concepts concerning computer-aided diagnosis; and these are outlined in Table 1. It is not helpful to talk of computers doing diagnosis at the present time, what is more useful is a system designed to aid the clinician in his own decision making performance. This implies that the system must be orientated towards the clinician and not centre around the computer. Adequate preparation is essential and most previous systems have probably failed because of the lack of preparation. This applies to the computer also; for most people aquire a computer and then try and find a use for it. The reverse should be the case - namely one should set out design criteria and then find a system which fits these criteria. Finally, any system should be evaluated in routine clinical practice.

Table 1

Fundamental Concepts of Computer-Aided Diagnosis and Decision-Making

1. Computer-<u>aided</u> diagnosis, not computer diagnosis.
2. Orientation towards clinician.
3. Adequate preparation essential.
4. State design criteria, <u>then</u> acquire hardware.
5. Evaluate in routine clinical practice.

METHODS OF COMPUTER-AIDED DIAGNOSIS

As indicated previously, adequate preparation is essential. As an illustration of this we in Leeds spent three years defining the problem, defining clinical categories and collecting a large amount of information on a structured basis from a series of 600 cases. This work is tedious but absolutely necessary, because unless the problem is studied in this depth at the onset, no computer system will be able to aid the clinician.

In assisting the clinician with his own decision making process, again as already indicated, the system must work in routine clinical practice. As an example, in our own system the patient comes into the ward and information is obtained from him by various doctors as part of a routine "clerking" process. This information is recorded on a special form (the design of which took one year and several observer variation trials). From here the information must be coded and entered into the computer. The computer then compares the information concerning the new case with that concerning 700 cases already in its memory, using a variant of Bayes' Theorem. The turn-round time from data entering to print-out of probabilities varies, but is at most 5 minutes. The print-out includes a copy of the patients case history, a set of probabilities (based on the conditional probabilities in the 700 cases already in the computer memory), and an analysis of the computers own record in diagnosing that disease over the past few years.

As far as hardware is concerned, again it is reasonable to refer to our fundamental concepts in Table 1; we initially began with a large and now obsolete computer costing £250,000. Only some two years later did we realise that the same work could be done on a desk-top machine costing 1% of the large computer price and capable of being operated by virtually anyone in the department. This illustrates that we should at the start of our study have studied design criteria rather than attempting to hang a system on to an already existing computer.

RESULTS

The only way in which to evaluate any computer-aided decision-making system is in routine clinical practice and we have been fortunate to be able to do this. We have analysed now just short of 10,000 cases, at a rate of approximately 250 per month. As regards the acute abdomen, the area in which we have most experience, we have carried out a prospective, consecutive, unselected, real-time, real-life trial between 1971-1973 on a series of 552 cases. In this the diagnosis of various doctors and the computer prediction was noted, in all instances before the patient went to the operating theatre. The results show an accuracy ranging from 40% when the patient was first seen to 81% for the most senior clinician to see each patient. Using the same data and making its decision before the patient went to theatre, the accuracy of the computer was 91%.

There are some potential criticisms to be levelled at the study and they are important. First the system may be person specific in that other people might not be able to use it. Second, the computer may not be necessary in that it may be possible to achieve the same accuracy with weighted tables or rules. Third, decision-making matters rather than accuracy of diagnosis. Finally, geographical variation in presentation may invalidate the results if an attempt is made to use the system elsewhere.

In attempting to remedy these defects we have used the system with a number of other clinicians and found comparable accuracy results - though there is quite clearly a need for a training period of a month or two before the clinicians learn the system. Weighted tables and rules have not in our hands been successful, but on the other hand we have found that decision-making and diagnosis are inextricably linked. It seems to us that the crucial question will come with the problem of geographical variation. How well will such systems work when transposed from one geographical area to another? Initial results indicate that our own system "travels" quite well but considerably more research is needed in this sphere.

Incidentally it might be mentioned that the effect of the computer-aided system on doctors appears to be beneficial. During our use of such a system we have noted considerable improvement in the doctors own performance. This may stem from the need to collect structured data as opposed to the very haphazard case history - or it may stem from the feed-back which the doctor gets from the computer.

CONCLUSIONS

All that one can say at the present time is that computer-aided diagnosis is feasible, potentially useful and effective.

It remains to be seen whether the sort of results obtained in our hands in assisting clinicians to make their own decisions and diagnosis can be obtained in different areas and different clinical spheres. If this is the case computer-aided decision making may well be one of its most useful applications in medicine. If not then it will remain - and perhaps rightly so - an esoteric pastime.

THE LONDON HOSPITAL COMPUTER SYSTEM — A CASE STUDY

W. Abbott

North East Thames Regional Health Authority

Management Services Division, St. Faith's Hospital
Brentwood, Essex

INTRODUCTION

In presenting this case study of the computer system at the London Hospital I should first explain that I left the London to take up the post of Regional Management Services Officer in the North East Thames Regional Health Authority last July. However, as Management Services Officer, I am still involved with the project, albeit at one stage removed, and when John Rowson, the present project director, was unable to come here today, I felt I could reasonably accept the invitation to speak for the project.

I am sure that you will all appreciate that it is not possible to cover all the aspects of a computer project that is of such a scale and complexity as that being developed at the London Hospital in just 30 minutes. There have been a large number of papers presented (both nationally and internationally), whole day seminars, and even a book has been devoted to the project. The subjects covered have ranged from the technical aspects of hardware and software to the user reactions, problems of privacy and so on. Today therefore I am going to content myself with presenting an overview of the project, indicating some of the salient features and pointing to some of the lessons that may have been learnt.

THE BEGINNING

As some of you may know the London Hospital was a pioneer in medical computing and had a well established and successful computer installation some ten years ago. As a consequence of this experience a number of ideas as to how computing might develop had already been expressed in 1967 when the D.H.S.S. began to establish its experimental programme. The London Hospital were invited to participate in this programme and the project was officially launched in 1968 on what some people have unkindly called the most appropriate date, 1st April.

Probably the earliest lesson in computing that had been learnt at the London was the necessity to provide for a multi-disciplinary approach to major problems and that a high level involvement was essential to success. In the case of the proposed real time system it was felt that from the earliest possible time the formation of a tightly knit, dedicated working group to drive the project was a prime need. Accordingly, even before the official launching of the project the group that subsequently became known as the Computer Executive was formed. It comprised a consultant physician, a senior nursing officer, the deputy house governor, the Director of O.R. and myself as the computing manager. This group had many years experience at the London, knew and trusted each other, and were all quite convinced as to the value of computers in the hospital environment. The project was also fortunate in that the group remained together, with but one change in 1972, from 1967 until quite recently.

THE PHILOSOPHY

The philosophy of approach and the resultant key decisions were evolved after many discussions both within the Executive and with the various interested groups in the hospital. Fairly obviously, the earliest decision was that concerning where the system should start. There were two basic courses open, one to develop a total computer system within a ward and then transfer other wards as and when possible; the second to develop a function across the hospital and then add more functions as and when possible. At that time, there was no experience that we could draw on either here in the U.K. or anywhere else. Consequently, we referred to our experiences of the introduction of other systems in the hospital and concluded that the problems of dual systems were such that they were best avoided. This together with other disadvantages decided the issue that we should opt for the establishment of a system function by function and we used the phrase horizontal development.

The next problem was to identify the first function. It happens that the London has a rather large out-patient department with total annual attendances of over three quarters of a million. In spite of the enthusiasm of the Executive it was felt that the sheer size of the files etc. was rather daunting and it was decided to concentrate first on functions associated with in-patients. It was considered that the first function to be developed should be waiting list followed by admission/discharge procedures. While there were some benefits to be obtained from these applications, they were principally being considered as enabling measures for the next functions where it was considered greater benefits could be obtained. These next functions were to be much more concerned with patient services and after much deliberation, the requesting and reporting procedures for laboratory services were selected. A major factor in formulating the decision was that a survey had demonstrated that over 70% of all in-patients had at least one laboratory test. Clearly any benefits obtained would be widespread and would hopefully be more easily identified. One other factor that also should be mentioned is that the hospital had already laid plans to obtain a small laboratory computer and it was expected that this would facilitate the transference of results to the main real time system. These then were the applications that were settled as constituting the first major system.

The next major decision concerned the method of communication to be available to the user in the real time system. As part of the overall philosophy of the system it had been agreed that the user should be in direct contact with the computer; that is, as far as possible there should be no intermediate step of specialised staff neither to code or prepare computer documents, nor to operate the terminals. It was agreed that the manual system largely provided this direct contact and that any intermediate stage would constitute an additional overhead that would tend to outweigh the possible benefits. Certainly, the introduction of such a stage would tend to make the system that more difficult to sell to the staff. Having established the concept the problem was to decide on the type of terminal and the method of use. The usual terminal at this time was the teletype but this was clearly too noisy and too slow. The answer proved to be the visual display unit using a tree branching technique. This technique uses a series of displays commencing with a standard screen offering a numbered list of available services. The selection of a number from the list provides the next screen with a further list of choices. Further selections are made until the required action from the computer is displayed precisely and this can be accepted and activated.

Using this technique compares well with manual systems; an example being that of filling in a request for a laboratory test. This involved the completion of a form on the ward by a doctor and took a minimum of 20 seconds. The maximum number of frames needed in tree-branching is five and takes only 15 seconds to complete. Thus the objective of the new system requiring no greater effort than the old could be achieved while the advantages of accuracy and legibility could be gained. It should perhaps be stated that the benefits to be gained on input would not be immediately available to the person involved in making the entry and it was very important to be able to demonstrate that extra effort for input of data was not necessary.

Having made these key decisions the next problem involved the selection of the actual computer. Here the London were required by the D.H.S.S. to give all manufacturers an opportunity to tender, although it was known that there were probably only 7 or 8 that could be expected to be able to supply the appropriate equipment. After some preliminary discussions (skirmishes might be a better word!) with some manufacturers, the Computer Executive drew up a draft invitation to tender. Effectively, it stated the requirements of the system that the Hospital was envisaging and specified items such as record sizes, file sizes, transaction rates, numbers of terminal sites, back-up requirements, maintenance requirements, software, etc., etc.

These specifications were summarised first in certain minimum requirements that tenders had to satisfy and second by certain desirable features that would gain preference for the tender that included such features.

Thus the hospital was setting out the system that was required and inviting the manufacturers to supply from their own range of equipment the best configuration for the job. In this way it was hoped that the Hospital would obtain the best possible buy.

Computer consultants were used to check this draft invitation to tender, and after considering their advice, and after discussions with the D.H.S.S. Computer branch, the document was issued. There followed a very hectic few months in which the number of possible suppliers was considerably cut back. Probably the most difficult task at this time was to convince the various manufacturers that the Hospital was genuinely in the open market, and would take the best offer.

The next stage was the evaluation of the tenders. Here again the Computer Executive called in consultants to check on a proposed course of action and, after some delays, eventually the Univac tender was successful.

One other aspect that was decided at what might be called the philosophy stage was that there should be an evaluation of the overall project. This was in association with the D.H.S.S. who were trying to obtain proof of the value of this type of computing to major hospitals. It is important to note that this evaluation was to be and is separate from the project control although there is close collaboration of course.

IMPLEMENTATION

Preparation for the introduction of the computer system began at a very early stage, indeed it can be said that the hospital was involved at the very beginning of the project. Formally, the medical and nursing members of the Executive were each supported by official committees of their colleagues, who provided advice on different aspects of the project as required. Generally, however, the Executive set out to provide a continuous programme of seminars, lectures, demonstrations and so on to all the staff of the hospital. In this way information about the project was disseminated and a running dialogue maintained between the Hospital and the project.

The process began even before the invitation to tender had been sent to the manufacturers when the Executive invited small groups of senior staff-consultants, senior nurses and administrators to day-long seminars on the project. These seminars took the form of a half day on the appreciation of computer techniques followed by another half day on the project. Effectively the time spent on the project in the early seminars was a discussion in which the ideas and concepts of the Executive were tested. Many contributions were made by the senior staff and gradually the project became more firm and the hospital knew that it was having a very large say in the directing of the whole system.

More seminars followed until virtually all senior staff had attended at least one full day and had ample opportunity to formally discuss the project with the Executive. Clearly, many informal discussions followed these seminars.

The next stage was to inform the next level of staff and use was made of study days, special talks, appreciation courses, etc. Of course many staff were already being directly involved with the systems analysts who were already classifying the current systems.

In March 1971 the computer was delivered and by the autumn it was necessary to start wiring up for the communication system. At this point then, it was necessary to start making our presence known to the ward staff. A demonstration program was devised for the V.D.Us. and as each ward was fitted with its V.D.U. the appropriate ward staff were shown the demonstration and invited to use the terminal when the system was live. This period was for two hours every day and enabled the hardware to be fully tested as well as stimulate the interest of the ward staff. These procedures were followed for all the thirty wards and the several departments where the V.D.Us. were sited.

As the settling-down of the equipment proceeded and the familiarisation programme was progressing, the first application was being prepared. This was the waiting list element of the admission discharge procedures, and the method of setting up of the existing manual file on the computer was under consideration. The choice basically was whether to prepare the file as a batch operation, or whether to use the two hours a day when the system was live for testing as an opportunity to build up the file in real time. The latter alternative was considered more attractive since the method had a number of particular advantages. First, the clerical staff were able to operate the system of entry to the waiting list without being under pressure and could build up confidence. Second, the application programmes could be thoroughly tested. Third, the wards could begin to experience what the live system would be like. Finally, the overall system (hardware and software) would be that much more tried and tested.

Thus the choice was made and the file was built up over 3 to 4 months. Then the application was taken live and the full waiting list suite of programmes was implemented, with very little problem at all.

The next application was that of the remaining procedures of the admission and discharge systems. It was expected that this would be a much more difficult implementation since the application affected all wards and several departments directly. Accordingly it was arranged that implementation teams would be used to instruct and support the ward staff over the introductory period. The concept was that the teams would be allocated to particular wards so that from the time the system went live at least one person from the implementation team would be available to each pair of wards the whole time the system was up (14 hours a day). This stage was to last two weeks, then the cover was to be reduced to one man per four wards for two weeks and finally one man per eight wards for two weeks.

Confidence was truly established by this plan, although in the event the teams were all completely withdrawn after just two weeks. It could be said that the project 'overkilled' the implementation but it is certain that the whole procedure had several good features. First, the implementation teams were formed from largely non-computer staff. This obviously was a most valuable mixing of hospital and computer staff. Second, the computer application team were able to concentrate on the program problems and the central admission office, without the distraction of problems from the wards. Finally there was the sure knowledge of back-up in depth for the introduction period.

With the admission/discharge system fully live there was a period of bug-chasing and settling down. Then the next step was to implement the first stage of the laboratory procedures. This was the requesting and reporting of microbiology tests. On this occasion it was not felt necessary to assemble a large implementation team since the wards were now very familiar with the basic principles involved in using the V.D.Us. Instead implementation consisted of an induction session for laboratory and ward staff during the two weeks prior to the date of going live. The application team then provided direct support for the following few weeks - primarily to the laboratory.

Requesting procedures for the remaining laboratories followed as the next application and the individual reporting procedures have followed one by one.

QUESTIONS ANSWERED

Thus there is now a genuine real-time system functioning as normal routine and an integral part of the hospital. Probably three major questions have already been answered by the system. First, when the project was mooted, it was not known if such a system could be built, especially within the financial constraints set. There were problems of hardware and software but these were all overcome and the system availability overall has been highly satisfactory and well within the standards originally set.

Second, in order to gain full benefits from the real time system it was essential that the staff should use the terminals freely and easily, without the need for special training. After the initial introduction of the system, there has been little need to mount special seminars etc. New staff are informed about the system as part of the normal induction procedures and there seems little problem in the operation of the terminals. This applies almost regardless of grade or profession - ward clerks, nurses, doctors, technicians, porters, all cope with the terminal with little more difficulty than the telephone.

The third question that has been answered is whether the system would be credible to the users. Would it be used and relied upon or would it be by-passed by the staff as so many hospital systems are, whether manual or computer. Again it would seem the answer is yes. Staff do rely on it; they complain,

they wish it would do more and more quickly, they raise the roof
on the odd occasion when the system breaks down or is late starting
or closed down early. Probably the last comment is the most
indicative of the positive answer to the question - as any
computer man will tell you - he knows his users are satisfied
when they complain about any withdrawal of service.

Whether the system can be economically justified is still
not proven. The project evaluation has identified a number of
savings and benefits but the full evaluation is not yet complete.
Subjectively, however, there is no doubt that the staff prefer
the system.

PROBLEM AREAS

Finally I would like to refer briefly to current problems
and disappointments. Probably the biggest disappointment is that
the time scales for getting applications live remain obstinately
long - too long. We must get from system design to implementation
faster. Various software and hardward tools to achieve this
purpose for real-time systems are in the pipe line but the
problem has still to be solved.

We still haven't got the right file structures and data base
systems generally don't produce fast enough response times. Stoke,
Birmingham and The London are probably near the point where better
structures could be defined.

Third, real time systems based on single processors, are very
difficult installations to run and develop. The initial systems
are of course relatively straight-forward from this point of view
but successive applications become increasingly difficult to
systems test to the required level. Birmingham, I believe, have
succeeded in providing for some testing underneath the real-time
system - using more core of course - and this may be an answer.
But there are also the problems of standby and maintenance for as
I have already indicated, as the hospital gets used to a real-time
system there arises a growing intolerance to anything less than a
100% service.

I think I have said enough about the project at the London to
indicate the scope, intent and to some degree the results achieved.
I am certain that this sort of computer service has its part to
play in the future of the N.H.S. side by side with other developments in the computer field.

TOWARDS MICROFILM SYSTEMS IN THE HEALTH SERVICE

E.J.Steadman

Managing Director, Old Delft (England) Ltd.

16, Barclay Road, Croydon, CRO 1JN

Abstract

With rapidly increasing costs of labour, in the future we shall be forced to accept automatic retrieval systems for all hospital records, including case notes, during the next ten or twenty years.

The considerable progress which has been made in storage of X-ray film copies over the last five years, has paved the way to a consideration of how other records can be stored and retrieved in smaller and more convenient forms, so that the ultimate, of all records being immediately and remotely retrievable in consulting rooms, clinics and wards, is rapidly becoming a practicability. For some records, conventional computer type storage and retrieval is not ideal, particularly where records are in pictorial form. For such records, a new type of microfilm storage would seem to give great advantages, and is capable of being integrated with computer stored records of other types into a comprehensive record system.

There is clearly no long term future in such labour-intensive filing and retrieval systems as have been in common use, in a society where labour is rapidly becoming the most costly raw material, and provision of the vast volume of space required is almost equally costly. This paper has arisen in an attempt to put forward less labour intensive systems and is the result of consideration of X-ray filing systems, which have been probably the most costly and cumbersome of hospital records in the past.

Over the last few years, X-ray film miniaturisation systems have been developed which enable the X-ray film in copy form to be included in the case notes, thus giving for the first time a fully comprehensive case record, which can be stored and retrieved as a single entity. Duplicate or master copies can additionaly be filed separately in a small department file in the X-ray department, so that the radiologist can refer to old films of a patient without the necessity of bringing the case notes, with their film copies into the X-ray department. The departmental filing envelope, containing X-ray request, report, and copy films is now becoming quite common. Such a record can equally, of course, form part of the master case note file very easily and then ironically, the X-ray record forms the smaller part of the standard case note file where once it was too large to be included therein.

Logically, therefore, the case note material should be further reduced in size, into a packet 8" by 6" or 20 cm. x 15 cm. Reduction of records to this size is by no means microfilming though it is a step in this direction, but it does have the advantage that such records can relatively easily be read with the naked eye, and therefore need no sophisticated read-out system. Such a case note packet has been designed for fully automated retrieval by a somewhat more sophisticated addition to a standard form of record file, fairly common in hospitals and certainly well known in other record environments.

Such a medical record system would be considerably less time consuming in filing and retrieval time, and considerably less space consuming than the present systems in general use. However, such a system would still basically be a manual system, once the miniaturised case note package has been identified, and for the long term even more reduction in labour content will almost certainly be necessary.

Clearly, computer storage of case notes is an attractive concept, since such a computerised record system would have the facility of providing a visual record on a screen, as well as the ready provision of a hard copy when desired for permanent local record, or communication with another hospital. And, without much doubt, the secrecy involved in computer storage, properly controlled, would certainly be no less than that provided by our present case note packets, which if my information is to be relied upon, quite regularly go astray even without deliberate intent, and at best are for the better part of their lives, both in and out of the file, in the charge of non-medical personnel, including those lay persons who are responsible in many cases for their transport from medical records department to clinic. Indeed, the dangers of secrecy in a computerised record system seem to have been dramatically over-emphasised in comparison with present systems.

Computer systems, with greater or less secrecy provisions, are becoming fairly common now in hospitals, though none to my personal knowledge has been established to provide the complete medical case note record. However, a computer type record is, to my mind, not the ideal for a comprehensive medical record, since it does not provide good facilities for storing pictorial matter, such as an X-ray picture or a photograph taken as a record of patient's condition.

Let us consider this aspect, which is an important one if a computerised type of medical record is to become a possibility.

If I am right in my contention that a computer does not store pictorial matter very well, (other than fairly simple line drawings, perhaps), we should consider other picture storage devices. In general, and in the context in which we are considering them, the filing and display of still pictures, we have only two practical systems, either magnetic or photographic. Taking magnetic recording first; my contention regarding inadequacy of computers for pictorial storage really stems from quite long experience of magnetic picture recording systems, both video tape and video disc. Since computer storage itself is done mainly by these methods, it suffers at least from the same limitation, and also quite a serious additional limitation, in that digitising the record must involve a considerable distortion of contrast range, apart from band-width limitation of resolution.

Turning to the systems which have been developed specifically for storage of images on magnetic tape, one major limitation is the considerable area of tape required to provide a single picture of good quality. If we take the medium quality 1" wide tape as an example, the total area for storage of one field of a T.V. picture (containing only half of the information in a complete picture) is close to 10 square inches, or around 10" length of tape, and double this would be required for a complete picture of medium definition. Similarly, the video disc provides a cumbersome storage medium and one which demands, for immediate retrieval, one record/replay unit per disc. Though it is more suited to storage and replay of still pictures than tape, one record unit using one replay disc which could store only some 200 pictures would be quite out of the question for our purpose. Better to use a modified video tape recorder for this purpose, since our present large reel of video tape could certainly store three to five thousand reasonable quality pictures, consisting of two interlaced fields. But even this would demand a very large number of record/replay units for any X-ray or medical illustration store.

However, the ultimate resolution obtainable with even quite sophisticated closed circuit television and magnetic recording, falls short of the best detail obtainable on an X-ray film or film copy, and this would clearly limit the ultimate usefulness of such an archival system.

The alternative, to use a photographic method of storage, brings us to the possibility of microfilm storage of patient notes, charts, photographs and X-ray films.

Microfilm storage systems have long been available for documents, and the use of a microfilm copy of an X-ray film has become quite commonplace, for the 6-year archival store. It is questionable, however, whether the information content of the microfilmed X-ray image, produced with relatively unsophisticated equipment, is adequate for our purpose, where the record would need to be adequate for comparison purposes almost from the moment after the film had been reported. And certainly, the retrieval of one particular frame from the larger number of reels of microfilmed copies which provide the archival X-ray store of many hospitals is time consuming and involves more labour and equipment than dealing with large size X-ray films.

Modern methods of microfilm filing and retrieval are now available which lend themselves well to our present purpose. The Kodak Retnar system of microfilmed X-ray images, is one such, where each image is fitted into its own record card, which can contain information from the radiologist's report, and the X-ray image itself can be retrieved by optical projection or a television viewing system.

However, for an integrated system where retrieval of case notes as well as pictorial information is done remotely, such a combined record card and X-ray microimage is not ideally practical.

Recently, a form of large microfiche store has been developed, which would appear to provide much of what is required for easy filing and retrieval of pictorial information, side by side with computer storage of notes and written reports.

This new system of microfilm storage uses the same general principles of retrieval as a programmed magnetic store typewriter – the storage of information being on plates which are stacked in the magazine store, and selected individually and positionally for read out of the information.

A small number of pilot installations of this type of file are presently being built for industrial filing purposes. These installations are mainly novel in respect of the filing and retrieval arrangements, since the actual microfilming of information employs relatively standard but good quality camera units, and the location of the microfilm "chip" in the microfiche is carried out in a conventional manner.

The large microfiche which forms the main storage element of the system will hold 300-16 mm. microfilm images, and might well be called a "macrofiche".

The 300,000 individual images, contained in 1000 of these "macrofiche" units in the filing system are retrieved simultaneously both optically on the viewing screen mounted within the file console, and by closed-circuit TV for remote viewing.

Each microfilm image, wherever located in the store, can be retrieved in less than one second (a typical retrieval of one image can be performed in 0.4 second), either by operation of the selection keys on the file console, or remotely from the remote viewing position. At the time of photographing the original information on to microfilm, its final position in the store is predetermined, and the film coded accordingly; it is then built into its correct position on its recorded macrofiche sheet, and this information stored in the computerised address store of the file. When subsequently recalled for retrieval this computer will instruct the retrieval mechanism in the shortest method of obtaining the required frame, which will then be retrieved for viewing in minimum time.

In addition to optical and TV viewing of the frame, a hard copy can also be prepared rapidly, for further detailed reference, posting to an outside agency or hospital or for filing in a temporary hard copy file.

Clearly this new system provides a nearly ideal adjunct to a computerised case note system, for dealing with charts, photographs, or X-ray film records.

This 16 mm system is designed to file microfilmed copies of documents of A4 size - roughly the size of a normal case note file. If it is adequate for reading typescript of this size, it is clearly adequate for most charts, and for many photographs which may be included in case notes, which, in general will be less than A4 in size, and therefore capable of better resolution on the final microfilm image.

The size of one filing console is such, as has been mentioned above, as to be capable of storage of 300,000-16 mm microfilm images. If used for storage of the whole of the case notes, this represents perhaps 10 to 15000 patients; but if used only for the "photographic" part of case notes, including X-ray film copies, some 50,000 patients' notes could be covered, with the remainder of the medical record stored in the computer store.

In cases where the maximum detail is required from the X-ray film record, it would be quite practicable for a special file to be provided, using macrofiches with 35 mm image size, each file then holding the equivalent of some 80,000 X-ray films. The photographic part of the record could still be contained in a 16 mm format store unit.

The possibilities of use of such a microfilm storage file are varied. As has been mentioned above it could be used for the entire case note files, though this would not seem an ideal method, as against a mixed system with computer storage.

One attractive possibility would be the use of the "Macrofiche" system to store a summary of the case notes, which would in many cases be adequate for subsequent reference. The original case notes, then, could well be stored in their original form, and would be called for on the few occasions when detailed examination of previous notes would be necessary. In such a system of summarised notes, a complete X-ray file could be stored in another cabinet store, so that, in addition to the summarised notes, the clinician could have immediate access to previous X-rays.

Again, there would be a choice of operating this special type of store either on line, or by a batch process. For the latter, hard copy would need to be provided in every case and for some purpose this might be the best method. However, it would seem that only an on-line system, where data is immediately retrievable on demand, would give the best utilisation of resources. Clearly in a situation where many departments of a hospital would need simultaneous access to stored material, some short time storage device would be necessary so that the clinician requiring the notes could examine them for an adequate period without preventing other departments from gaining access to the file. A suitable short time storage device could be provided in the form of a magnetic disc recorder, which could retain up to one hundred separate "pages" of information, including pictorial and X-ray matter, whilst the main store would be free to transmit data to other departments. Such a system has been described before for an X-ray storage and retrieval of this general type, however it could very well be used for any microfilmed data.

This paper has outlined some of the possibilities which present technology opens to us for filing systems which can be operated with the minimum of labour. Such systems could today be assembled and then only would we be able to evaluate their usefulness in practice. They would, of course, be capital intensive, but not necessarily any more costly over a number of years as compared with our present labour-intensive systems of filing case notes and medical records of all types.

MULTI-IMAGE STORAGE

J. Hambleton

Chemical Electronics (Birtley) Ltd.
Hutton Close
Crowther Estate
Washington
Tyne and Wear U.K.

Utilising the linear storage capabilities of film, it is possible to store a number of overlapped exposures on a single frame and subsequently retrieve the individual images.

Multiple imagery comprises three general operations:-

Spatial encoding.

Linear Storage.

Optical demodulation.

The concept of multiple imaging can be explained by considering its radio analogue. Although radio signals are broadcast simultaneously from many separate sources, the radio receiver has the ability to discriminate between signals, isolate that signal required, demodulate and reproduce the original sounds of the broadcast. While one radio signal appears very much like another, the carrier frequency which it modulates is unique to one particular radio station. The radio receiver tuner filters the broadcast band, permitting only the desired frequency to pass.

In the optical counterpart the sound amplitude varying with time is transposed to a variation of light intensity across the image of a scene.
Modulating of a light image is simply done by placing a black and white grating in front and very close to the front of a film in a camera. The periodic black bars in the grating restrict light falling on the emulsion, which after development results in a modulated carrier on the film, (Fig. 1.)

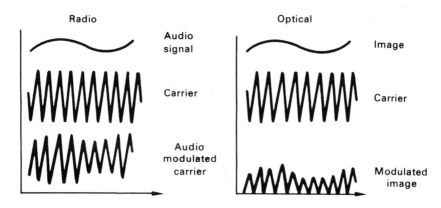

Fig. 1. Modulation of an Image.

The requirement is to store more than one image on the same film and yet separate them. In the radio case the secret lies in the use of different carrier frequencies. In the optical case a carrier frequency is used in which the light amplitude varies with the distance across the film. Unique optical modulation will be created if either the periodicity of the grating or its angular direction is changed. Rotating the grating through 90°, makes it possible to allow a second exposure on the same piece of film: this exposure will have a modulation at right angles to the first. Projecting such a film will result in the display of a double exposure and a 'tuner' is required to filter out one of the images and pass only the desired image.

It is necessary to digress at this point and discuss some aspects of diffraction. If collimated light derived from a point source in the back focal plane of a lens is passed through a second lens, at a distance equal to the focal length of the second lens a spot of light is formed, which is the image of the source. Placing a grating in the collimated beam replicates the point image which becomes a series of spots in a line perpendicular to the direction of the grating slits, (Fig. 2). The brightest spot is the centre one and is known as the zero or dc order. The diffraction orders decrease in intensity outward from the zero order; they are referred to as the first order, second order etc. The spacing between spots is directly proportional to grating frequency, focal length of the objective lens and the illuminating wavelength. Although each spot contains all of the information of the original spot, it is no longer an image of the light source but a complex convolution of the light source image and diffraction grating spectrum. The image of the grating has undergone a Fourier transformation and the plane at which these spots appear is known as the Fourier transform plane.

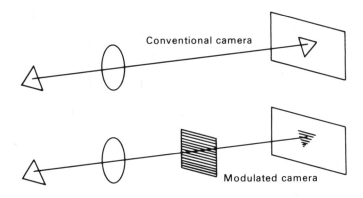

Fig. 2.

Considering the double exposed transparency in which each scene is modulated in a different direction, we have basically a complex grating in two directions, replacing the simple grating in the optical system shown in Fig. 2, with the transparency, results in two sets of diffraction orders at the Fourier transform plane. Allowing only the central or zero order to pass through an aperture placed at the Fourier plane will display a double exposure since this order is common to both images. However, if we locate our aperture on either "arm" of the diffraction pattern, so that, say, the first order may pass, only one image will be seen on projection since the orders in that arm are unique to only that image. Moving the aperture to a similar order of the other arm, the first image is excluded and the second is displayed. The opaque screen which contains the aperture acts as a tuner as it rotates on the optical axis. Just as the radio broadcasts can be received by tuning to the frequency of transmission, optical images can be received by tuning to the direction of modulation.

Having considered the production of two images, there is no reason why one cannot consider storing a greater number simply by rotating the grating in the camera. Rotating the grating every $18°$ should produce ten images. The question now arises, "How many images can be stored?"

This can be answered by considering the effects at the Fourier transform plane. The image on a film can be defined as a density variation as a function of two spatial co-ordinates x and y (Fig. 3.)

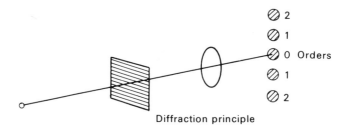

Diffraction principle

Fig. 3.

The Fourier spectrum of the image appears as a diffused spot of light with maximum brightness in the middle. In the diffraction, all low frequency information (areas where the density changes slowly) appears in the centre of the spot. The high frequency information (such as grass, fencing, venetian blind) exists at the edges of the spot. As the spots pass through an aperture, if that aperture diameter is too small, the edges of the spot will be clipped, resulting in a loss of high frequency information. Using a larger diameter aperture reduces the number of discrete positions in the 180 degree arc (Fig. 4.).

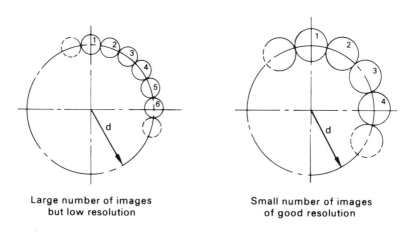

Large number of images
but low resolution

Small number of images
of good resolution

Fig. 4.

To specify the number of images to be stored it is first necessary to specify the resolution required for any one image. The resolution allowed by a given size aperture in frequency space is calculated simply.

MULTI-IMAGE STORAGE

In Fig. 5, the first diffraction order appears at a distance 'd' from the central order as a result of a grating carrier frequency of w1/mm, an aperture of diameter 'a' will allow a bandwidth in a one to one image of aw/d or an image resolution of aw/2d.

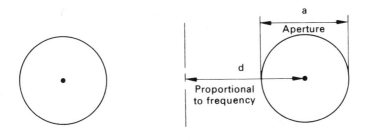

Fig. 5.

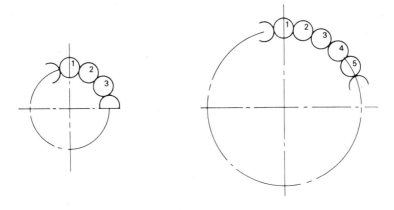

Fig. 6.

The second consideration is the maximum number of images to be stored. This entails consideration of the film resolution. Doubling the frequency of the grating doubles the distance of the first diffraction order from the central order. This in turn provides more room in frequency space to accommodate more discrete aperture positions (Fig. 6). For a given image resolution, increasing the carrier frequency increases the number of possible stored images.

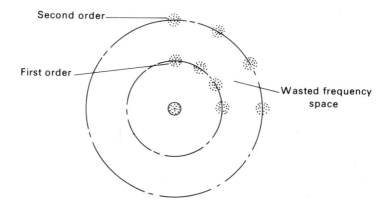

Fig. 7.

In order to double the grating frequency, however, the recording film must be able to record the modulation; otherwise no diffraction will occur. As a rule of thumb the resolution cut off of the film must be at least double the grating frequency.

So far the use of a simple grating has been considered and we have confined the use to the first diffraction order. However, the actual diffraction pattern consists of a number of orders as there is a band of wasted frequency space between the orders. This waste can be minimised by use of higher frequency gratings. One set of exposures can be produced by rotation of the first grating through 180 degrees, a second grating of higher frequency is then positioned in place of the first and another series of exposures taken. A further set can be taken with an even higher frequency grating and the major part of the frequency space can be used, (Fig. 8).

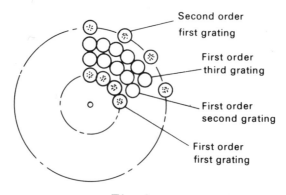

Fig. 8.

Using a single grating ten images can be adequately stored on half of a 35 mm frame of KODAK AHU microfilm with sufficient resolution on playback to be able to view alphanumeric information at x12 magnification on a viewing screen. Similar considerations with a microfiche (4 inch x 6 inch) at 3x magnification would allow the storage of 200 images if several gratings were used. Normal microfilm techniques usually store about half of this number and documents are reduced drastically in size 24x, 40x or even greater), because of the large reduction factor the associated optics must be of good quality and extremely rigidity mounted. Any speck of dust, will, on reconstruction, appear as a large blemish. As the images are closely packed the XY locator mechanism must be precisely made. Using multiple imagery far less reduction is required with resultant enhancement of image quality. As the magnification on reconstruction is far less, particles and scratches do not appear as large blemishes. Finally, the XY locator is replaced by a disc containing an aperture and rotates on the optical axis of the projector.

As the multiple images appear on the film as a mixed up jumble they cannot be read directly by the human eye and the information can be kept secret (an important factor in hospital records).

There is a limited ability to present animation from one frame of a picture. For example, a series of X-rays taken at intervals after an intravenous injection could each be photographed via the M.I. camera and by spinning the disc in the Fourier transform plane, the flow of the injected fluid could be observed.

A further extension of the technology is to use three coloured gratings and then reproduce excellent colour images from black and white films.

The author wishes to thank Dr. G.B. Parrent, Jnr., of Technical Operations Ltd., for providing the excellent information for the presentation of this paper.

PART VI

Ergonomic Contributions to Medical Diagnosis

CHAIRMAN'S INTRODUCTORY STATEMENT

Clive J. A. Andrews

Senior Lecturer in Ergonomics

Napier College, Edinburgh

Ergonomics is conceived as being composed of two inter linked components; one scientific, the other technological.

Ergonomics can be described as a multidisciplinary science which concerns itself with understanding what makes human beings tick and how the variability of individuals expresses itself in the special context of the work environment.

Its technological aspect is in the application of that knowledge so that people can cope successfully with the various elements which together with themselves comprise a system whose objectives are related to the performance of activities definable as work.

Thus Ergonomics seeks to study the following areas regarding people:

1. How they gather information from whatever the environment in which they must operate.

2. How they process information and take decisions.

3. How they respond to the decisions taken and to environmental inputs both overtly through motor actions and covertly through responses which are in the realm of the physiological, psychological and biochemical.

4. How the safety and health of individuals are affected by inputs from, or elements in the environment.

Applied Ergonomics with its emphasis on providing short term comfort as well as the eradication of those environmental features which lead to long term disability can clearly be regarded as a branch of preventive medicine.

This, the final session of the conference contains contributions from four speakers. Three of our speakers are experienced in applying ergonomics to their specialisms in the area of Medical diagnosis. The opening paper is presented by an Ergonomics specialist employed in Industry. He will indicate how the principles of Ergonomics as utilised by the Industrial Ergonomist can be beneficially applied to the concepts governing the approach to Medical Diagnosis.

INDUSTRIAL EXPERIENCE OF ERGONOMICS AS APPLIED TO CLINICAL

DIAGNOSIS

        G.J. Gillies

        Manager of Ergonomics
        Pilkington Bros. Ltd.
        St. Helen's, Merseyside U.K.

    Ergonomics is concerned with the practical study of the inter-relation between men, machines and environment.

    Experience over a wide field has shown that the failure to properly consider the man as an integral part of the system leads to ineffective systems. The main concern of the ergonomist in a basic manufacturing industry is the production system, since this is seen as the prime man/machine system. The basic approach is man centred, and this is a natural counterbalance to technology which tends to specify equipment and let the jobs take care of themselves afterwards. In the haste to computerise and to modernise, in some of our industries, certain designers have lost sight of the fact that it is people who control systems and processes. The modern equipment is often considered an end in itself. This has led to the alienation of the worker in Motor Industry and to the neglect of the quality of working life even though the standard of living has been rising.

    Well, what has this to do with the scientific aids to clinical diagnosis? I suggest it has a great deal.

    Firstly, the concept of the man centred approach seems extraordinarily apt since the clinician is controlling the treatment of peoples' health and well being. Secondly, the machines should be very carefully integrated into the clinical diagnosis system or team.

    Clinical diagnosis can be likened to classical fault finding where the faulty circuit or system demonstrates certain cues or symptoms to the maintenance operator. The correct interpretation of these cues, together with other tests made so as to isolate the cause or causes of failure, constitutes strategy. Independent of electronic technology (relays, transistors, solid state). Figure 1 shows that localising and isolating the fault takes longer than rectifying. Table 1 gives the diagnosis time for different types of equipment. In clinical treatment the situation is much more complex since there is a continuous interaction between diagnosis and treatment.

The training method consists of providing people with the basic skills and information to do the job and then teaching them correct procedures by stating fail symptoms and noting the strategies adopted. The work of Dale, and repeated by ourselves, shows that certain people are more 'logically' structured in their thoughts and approach than others. Hence behaviour can be classified as optimal repetitious or redundant at any given time. Table 2 gives the general results. The point is that each test taken in the fault diagnosis should add information and that the next move should take account of all previous moves. Actions are also influenced by the circuit configuration. People tend to go towards the junction points initially. In a similar way the clinician may be more attracted by certain aspects of the patients symptoms.

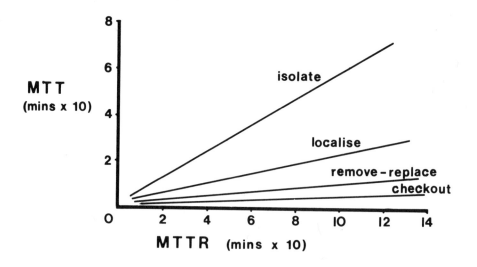

Fig. 1. Maintenance Task Time (MTT) versus Mean Time To Repair (MTTR) for modular-designed equipment

Table 1

Typical Diagnosis Times

TYPE OF EQUIPMENT	DIAGNOSIS TIME AS % OF TOTAL DOWNTIME	
Electronic	90	
Electrical	65	
Hydraulic	40	
Pneumatic	40	if simple
Mechanical	30	

Table 2

Operator Actions In Fault Finding

| CIRCUIT TYPE | ACTIONS % | | | AVERAGE TIME |
	Redundant	Helpful	Optimal	
Simple	13	76	11	15 s.
Complex	15	77	8	28 s.

In process control, we have found that there is a marked job knowledge difference between highly skilled foremen and less skilled operators. An interview approach was used. In addition, not all foremen could recall all the actions needed to overcome production faults, but that jointly they held most of the knowledge. The use of job aids was both logical and desirable. At this stage, it was evident that actions had to be ordered and some time scale indicated (strategy had to be constructed). Once again it was found that even skilled foremen would not always order their actions in the same sequence, and typically, only the first 1-4 actions could normally be placed in definite order. Following this, a non-structured cycling process or search process typically resulted.

The point I am making is that this is expected behaviour. Furthermore, the timing of actions could be markedly different for foremen with the same agreed sequence of actions purely because of personal traits.

I would suggest therefore, that clinicians with differing skills and experience presented with the same basic information will similarly not always draw the same conclusions.

In addition, the detailed information concerning specific diseases or ailments, whilst important, will not in itself ensure successful diagnosis. The same skilled foremen who had more detailed job knowledge were also able to perform a computer simulation more successfully than the less skilled operators. Figure 2 shows this. This result shows that the foreman also possessed a strategy superior to operators.

It is therefore the combination of job knowledge and strategy which distinguishes a skilled process operator or trouble shooter from the less skilled operator. I would respectfully suggest the same could be true of junior doctors and consultants. In addition to all this, we have found that unless the jobs of each team member are fully integrated then production suffers. The same parallel could apply to the doctor-nursing teams.

The use of scientific aids to diagnosis must be complementary to the skills of the whole team. Simply stated, people are superior to machines for pattern recognition, detection of small signals against background noise (or important information from trivial) and for adaptability. The adaptability of people is difficult to quantify, but in most situations computer control can only cover part of the total range of alternatives. People are not good monitors, or in reliably performing routine repetitive work. The role of the equipment should be to reduce unnecessary repetitive work and to provide a monitoring role. The specification of the hardware requirements should preferably take place

INDUSTRIAL EXPERIENCE OF ERGONOMICS

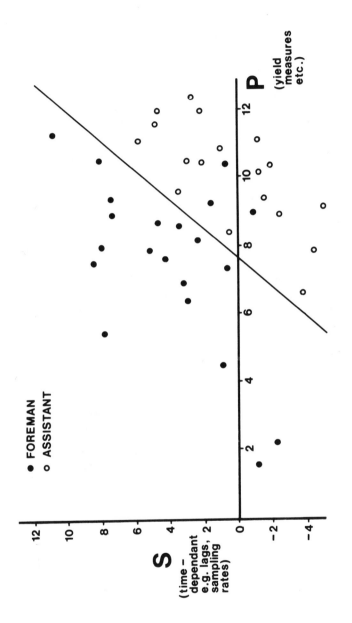

Fig. 2. Performance vs. Strategy Components

only after allocation of functions between staff and machines.

There are several points to raise once machines become predominant in the clinical diagnosis. Firstly, there will be a tendency to lose the skills associated with the tasks taken over by the machines. Secondly, the clinician and the team must understand the role and limitations of the machine. The machine complexity will also dictate the maintenance skills required and this has also to be carefully considered.

In addition, the very presence of machines may modify clinical diagnosis procedure. It may result in patients being wired up to the machine by junior staff and some initial diagnosis made before the senior clinician becomes involved. There may be a tendency to use the machine in more circumstances than is warranted just like the misuse of computers by some specialist subject users found by a recent study by HUSAT, Loughborough. I have of course deliberately over-emphasised this point to create an awareness of parallel situations which have already occurred in industry.

The link between the clinician and the scientific aids to diagnosis can be described as the man-machine interface. Typically, if too much information is presented to people, an over simplication of the information is made. If information is presented in a visual display unit instead of providing data or complex traces, certain key parameters should be presented in the form of a symmetrical pattern. This enables the observer to detect a deviation from 'normal' as quickly as possible. This has been emphasised by Wolff and others, see Figure 3. However, this implies that the parameter sensitivities are fairly well known with respect to the patients state of health. When the sensitivities are clearly established, then automatic alarms can be used. A difficulty can arise if alarms are too finely set, since experience of computer aided control rooms and railway accidents show that frequent false alarms lead to a tendency to ignore all alarms. Also the time taken to respond to a change of state of certain body functions may have a crucial result to the patient's well being. Can a machine with its associated transducers placed on the patient always respond adequately, or is the clinician much better? This may well depend on particular situations.

The use of computers to analyse traces and information, leads to operational problems which could cause delay in diagnosis if data entry has to be batched. The use of such techniques to assist diagnosis must be assessed with regard to the likely effect of the delay on the patient's health. This time constraint on data processing is experienced by industry when scheduling orders.

INDUSTRIAL EXPERIENCE OF ERGONOMICS 249

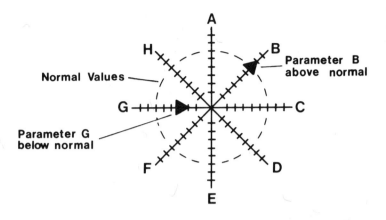

Fig. 3. Wolffs Polar Diagram

Returning to one of my earlier points, the strategy adopted by the clinician in the use of the equipment and his own procedures will be a crucial determinant in successful diagnosis. In industry, perceptual information is an important input to the process operator and a skill often difficult if not impossible to automate out. Similarly the clinician will no doubt be making careful visual observations of the patient which will interact with the other information to form the diagnosis.

It is apparent that one should ensure that the combination of the scientific aids to diagnosis and the clinical team is balanced. Secondly, that training should equip each team member or the individual with all the necessary knowledge and skills associated with the patient and the back up equipment.

Finally, I feel that strategy is bound to play an important part in clinical diagnosis and treatment. Since strategy is a longer-term acquired skill, it follows that special attention should be paid to the development of strategy in staff training. This has been done by flow chart techniques for product fault situations in industry. These are constructed by those most experienced. Also, one must recognise that strategies sometimes need modifying and that careful record and analysis of strategies and their effectiveness provides the feedback of information.

THE RATIONALE OF CLINICAL PROBLEM SOLVING

Donald L. Crombie

Director, Royal College of General Practitioners
Lordswood House, Lordswood Road, Harborne
Birmingham B.17. 9DB

Modern medical care systems become ever complex but their main purpose remains unchanged. That <u>purpose is to help individuals solve or ameliorate their clinical problems while maintaining maximal social competence</u>. Conventional clinical problems are those of which the patient is aware and for which he initiates the problem solving process. Increasingly, medical care systems under pressure from society, are extending this narrower purpose to include presymptomatic detection and to extend the strategy of prevention wherever possible. I shall be focussing here on conventional clinical problem solving partly because this is still the main area of activity of the system and partly because good clinical assessment strategies incorporate the useful presymptomatic diagnostic and preventive procedures as their relevance is demonstrated (1).

In fig.i (adapted from Horder & Horder 1954) the average pattern of illness experience during a lifetime is schematically presented. Only $5\pm$ of the 100 episodes of illness brought to medical care can be classed as serious or life threatening. In Great Britain, practically all clinical problems including these five serious illnesses, are brought first to general practitioners as the primary assessors of previously undifferentiated clinical problems.

<u>The conventional diagnostic model</u>: The traditional model for this strategy (fig.ii) is based on the assumption that information from the symptoms and physical signs is elicited from the patient during the consultation. This information is then marshalled for the purpose of establishing a diagnosis.

Fig.i

MEDICAL CARE AND RECOGNISED ILLNESS

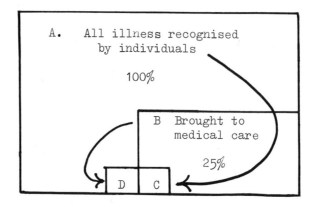

Normal illness Expectancy in Life
Number of Episodes

A   400
B   100
C   5 ±

C. Referred for Hospital Care
    1.5% ±

D. Hospital attendances without previous referral
    0.2%

C & D refer to Great Britain

Adapted from Horder & Horder (1954)

RATIONALE OF CLINICAL PROBLEM SOLVING

Fig.ii

CLINICAL PROBLEM SOLVING
TRADITIONAL PATHWAY

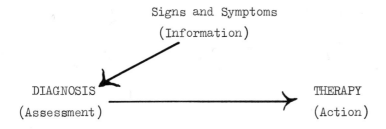

Fig.iii

ALTERNATIVE PATHWAY

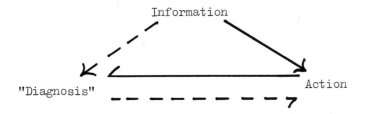

Once the problem is diagnosed, rational therapy can be implemented. However our patients present to us with clinical problems and these seldom equate on a one-to-one basis with any one individual diagnosis or disease process.

The elements of clinical problems: These elements can be classified as:
           physical ("organic"/structural);
           emotional and/or psychiatric and;
           social.

The relationships of these three elements are complex (Table I). For example, while 52% of the problems brought to general practitioners have no psychiatric element (other than the natural anxiety accompanying that physical illness), 48% have a psychiatric component which must be taken into account and in 27% this psychiatric element is as important or more important than the physical component,(2). The ratios for any social component are similar but they have a very different significance. More often than not, any social component in a clinical problem is simply the result of the prior physical or psychiatric morbidity and hardly ever the primary cause. Most problems then, are a complex mixture of two or even three separate diagnostic dimensions.

Diagnostic accuracy: How isomorphic or congruent are the diagnostic labels used by clinicians with the actual clinical problems? For primary care (Table II) just over half (3) the clinical problems are associated with a firm diagnosis and less than one-third with a tentative diagnosis or "best guess". For 8% of problems no diagnosis was made at all. In practical terms, the 6% classified as " eliminative diagnosis" are important in that the clinician can be certain that no serious or treatable illness is being missed while being quite uncertain of the true diagnosis (4) (5) (6).

Not only is isomorphism of the diagnostic label with the clinical problem poor but the information content of the actual labels is inadequate. For only 5% of the 500 morbid processes most frequently encountered by general practitioners and described by these labels, is the full aetiology and pathology established (3).

Alternative diagnostic strategies: Notwithstanding the poor information content of diagnostic labels and low level of accuracy with which they are used in practice, patients still have their problems adequately resolved and receive appropriate treatment. If this last statement is true it must be achieved by a decision making pathway (fig.3) which goes directly from signs and symptoms to therapy, from information directly to action. In this alternative model therefore, the choice of a "diagnosis" may be

TABLE I

The relationship of the organic, emotional and social components of clinical problems

	I	II	III	IV	V
Emotional/organic	52	21	13	6	8
Social/organic	48	32	10	1	9

Figures as percentage distributions are based on two separate sets of 100 representative clinical problems. The first set concerns any emotional content and the second set any social content. Each problem was assessed on the following scale:

I   A problem all or nearly all organic.

II   A problem mainly organic but with some abnormal emotional (or social) content.

III   A problem with organic and emotional (or social) content in equal proportion.

IV   A mainly emotional (or social) problem but with some organic content.

V   A problem all or nearly all emotional (or social).

Table II

DIAGNOSTIC ACCURACY

No diagnosis	8%
Tentative diagnosis	30%
Eliminative diagnosis	6%
Firm diagnosis	56%

Information content of diagnostic labels used in PRIMARY CARE.

For only 5% $\pm$ is there a generally agreed knowledge of aetiology and pathology.

RATIONALE OF CLINICAL PROBLEM SOLVING

determined more by the initial choice of action or therapy than vice versa.

This situation was explored in a paper by Howie (7). Respiratory infections account for 22.8% of the new diagnostic problems presenting to general practitioners. There are twelve commonly used diagnostic labels accounting for 18.4% (Table III) of all new episodes and a further 4.3% attributable to the remainder (8). There are more than 40 different symptoms or symptom complexes but only two important therapeutic alteratives. These are :-

To prescribe a broad spectrum antibiotic, or ;
no antibiotic.

There are four other subsidiary categories concerned with restrictions of activities. These are :-

No restrictions ;
Confine to house and therefore off work;
Confine to bed, or ;
Admit to hospital.

The twelve diagnostic labels fall into two groups. The five morbid processes in group A are "serious" while the remaining seven in group B are relatively trivial. The conventional diagnostic pathway (fig i) is more likely to be appropriate to conditions in group A and the alternative (fig ii) to conditions in group B.

Sixty percent (299) of the 502 patients in the study (Howie 1972)(7) received an antibiotic (Table IV). Compared with this basic rate, 93% of patients with positive chest signs, 99% of patients with "serious" diagnoses (group A) and only 45% of patients with "trivial" illnesses (group B) received antibiotics. Diagnoses in group A have a closer correlation with the use of antibiotics than has the presence of abnormal signs in the chest. However, 57% (192) of the 339 patients with no abnormal chest signs had no antibiotics compared with 55% (202) of those 368 patients with diagnoses in group B. There is a marginally better correlation therefore between "absent abnormal chest signs " and no antibiotic therapy than with a "trivial" diagnosis and no antibiotic therapy. The relative importance of the information from the presence or absence of chest signs is indicated by the differences in the ratios of (27 out of 38) 71% and 42% (139 out of 330) for correlations with use of antibiotics for patients with and without abnormal chest signs respectively when the diagnosis is trivial (group B). The corresponding ratios for patients with more "serious" diagnoses are 100% (125 out of 125) and 89% (8 out of 9). While the presence or absence of abnormal chest signs contribute maximum discrimination between alternative action in

TABLE III

DIAGNOSIS IN RESPIRATORY ILLNESS

GROUP A

("serious" illness)

Pneumonia
Acute Bronchitis
Tracheobronchitis
Bronchiolitis
Chest Infection

GROUP B

("Trivial" illness)

Coryza
Respiratory Tract Infection
Upper Respiratory Tract Infection
Influenza
Bronchial Catarrh
Pharyngitis
Tracheitis

(After Howie 1972)

TABLE IV

The Use of Antibiotics in Relation to Chest Signs in 502 patients with 12 specified respiratory diagnoses.

Illnesses (Grouped by seventy)	Chest Signs Positive			Chest Signs Negative			ALL patients
	Antibiotics			Antibiotics			
	+	−	Total	+	−	Total	
Group A	125	0	125	8	1	9	134
Group B	27	11	38	139	191	330	368
A + B	152	11	163	147	192	339	502

(After Howie 1972)

    60% ($\frac{299}{502}$) received antibiotics.

    93% ($\frac{152}{163}$) with positive chest signs, received an antibiotic.

    99% ($\frac{133}{134}$) with serious illness (A) received an antibiotic

    45% ($\frac{166}{368}$) with trivial illness (B) received an antibiotic.

However 57% ($\frac{192}{339}$) with negative chest signs had negative antibiotics compared with

    55% ($\frac{202}{368}$) with trivial illness (B) negative antibiotic.

In Group B { 71% ($\frac{27}{38}$) with positive chest signs had an antibiotic compared with

42% ($\frac{139}{330}$) with negative chest signs had an antibiotic.

In Group A { 100% ($\frac{125}{125}$) with positive chest signs had an antibiotic compared with

89% ($\frac{8}{9}$) with negative chest signs had an antibiotic.

patients given "trivial" diagnoses, the opposite is true for those given "serious" diagnoses. However the equivalent ratios of 100% and 89% indicate that even for "serious" diagnoses, considerable additional information is still involved. We can infer from these ratios that action for the treatment of relatively trivial illnesses is determined more by the presence or absence of abnormal chest signs than by the diagnosis ultimately reached. Even for "serious" conditions, the contribution of this important sign symptom complex is crucial.

The actual process of clinical decision making is however probably a step by step process. Information in the form of elicited signs and symptoms is from the onset, being related to a primary set of alternatives, "serious" or "trivial" and a secondary set of alternative "actions". While this is going on, actual alternative conventional "diagnoses" will be considered and tested by search for further information to refute them when any possible alternative is "serious" (9). Where no " serious " alternatives are generated by the process, the decision making relies more on the information inherent in the direct relationship of sign symptom complexes to action. Even where serious alternatives are a possibility, it is likely that decisions about appropriate action still have priority and influence the choice of any one "diagnosis" from the alternatives, quite as much as information from the sign/symptom complex directly.

Previously recorded data: In a study (10) of the "nature of information used in clinical decision making " by 50 general practitioners, it was shown that most of the information actually utilised for assessing new problems in primary care was generated de novo at the time of the consultation and could not have existed in any a priori record. At the same time, the information actually recorded in the past was seldom used or appropriate to the assessment of any new problem. The personal doctor interacting with his patient brings to the consultation a special type of a priori knowledge. In essence during his previous contacts with the patient he has accumulated information consisting of a general awareness of areas which might be of importance in the future. This generalised knowledge may relate to the patient's marital, social or work situation. For example, while visiting a patient at home with tonsillitis, the doctor may observe that the house is dirty, and that the wife is a slut. This information is irrelevant to the assessment of the present problem but some element of it may be of crucial importance in the assessment of some future problem. The awareness of relevant "nodal" areas (11) such as this, act as keys which can unlock when needed, data specific to some particular clinical problem when it arises.

These generalisations refer particularly to the 95 relatively trivial illnesses. For the $5^{\pm}$ serious illnesses during any one

RATIONALE OF CLINICAL PROBLEM SOLVING

individual's life, this is still true of the initial assessment. However the serious illnesses demand recurrent reassessments over time and appropriate record systems will now accumulate data which has a high probability of being useful in the future. The conventional ante-natal card used during a pregnancy is a good example. However once the pregnancy is completed, this detailed data is seldom relevant to the future, even to future pregnancies.

The clinical record: We can now consider the implication or the structure of appropriate records for primary care. The record for the 95 "trivial" illnesses generated during consultation with the patient will use information ad hoc to the problem (fig.iv) with low probability of existing in any a priori record. This ad hoc information will also have a low probability of usefulness for any future problems. Its purpose therefore is limited in time to initiating appropriate action. All such notes are therefore ad hoc to this process and have fulfilled any usefulness once this point is reached. Thereafter they can remain in an archive type record in the original manual form.

On the other hand a cumulative abstracted listing of "diagnoses" and therapeutic "actions" can form a higher level record, easily assessible in the patient's file. At a higher level still, can be a list of any serious illnesses and their treatments plus important "nodal" information.

The small proportion of serious, chronic illnesses such as hypertension, diabetes, cardiac failure, rheumatoid arthritis and cancer, require a special type of " flow-chart" record, ad hoc to the illness and specially designed. It is also true that the requirements of medical auditing are dictating much more systematisation of records than outlined here but we must be certain that the additional costs of any such further systematisation solely for this purpose are justified.

Information for clinical decision making: All primary assessment and the ultimate responsibility for integrating all continuing care, resides with the community or primary care team. This consists today of the general practitioner with district and other nurses, health visitors, social workers sometimes and appropriate secretarial and administrative staff. This team operates ideally from one appropriately designed Group Practice or Health Centre building (fig.v).

All information flow involved in clinical problem solving, has the community care team as its only universal node. This node is therefore the point at which selection and generalisation of data should rationally take place, the selection and generalisation being dictated by the functions of the secondary users in hospital and other settings. The only clinical information with any universal

Fig. iv

CONTENT OF RECORD

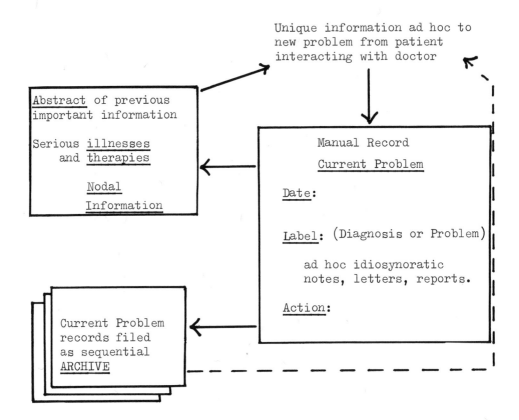

RATIONALE OF CLINICAL PROBLEM SOLVING

Fig. v

INFORMATION FLOW

(Clinical problems)

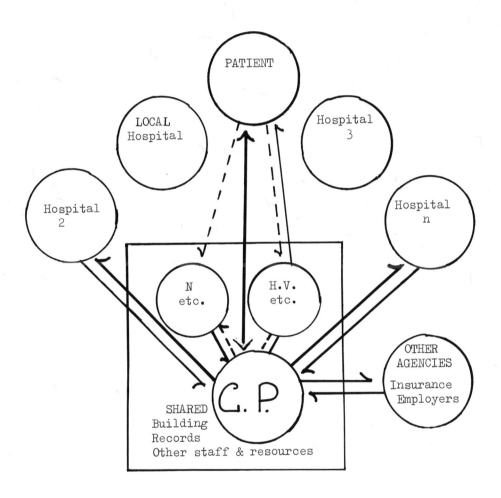

utility outside the team is the cumulative listing of serious illnesses and therapies. This applies to government agencies, insurance companies, employers, solicitors and other agencies outside the health service as well as to consultants and community physicians as our professional colleagues within the health service. Apart from this limited clinical information with universal utility and such data as the patient's name, address, age, sex, marital status and occupation, the structure of any communication from the primary users to other outside agencies is nearly always idiosynoratic and ad hoc to the patient's current problem. Because the primary record is used largely by the primary care team and only appropriate extracts or generalisations are needed for other purposes or by other professionals outside the team it can remain therefore in manual form.

Information for administration and planning: This review is specifically concerned with clinical problem solving and decision making. However a comment should be made about information for administrative and management purposes if only because the same general principles apply. Where maximum autonomy is given to the primary care team within its role as primary assessor and co-ordinator of continuing care, information by planners and administrators can be in the form of generalised statements of goal achievement and role fulfilment. For example if it is agreed that a reasonable aim for any immunisation programme among children is the completion of the programme for a minimum of 95% of children in the practice by a certain age, then only when this is not achieved, will management be interested in more detailed information.

It is also true however, that the administrative and management needs of the health service would be economically extended and improved by systematisation of non-clinical information. For example, automation of the Family Practice Committee procedures being explored now in model systems (13), may well be shown to have economic as well as more fundamental advantages over the present manual systems.

Summary and Conclusion:

Patients have _problems_.

Problems are a mixture of psychiatric/emotional, organic and social components.

Only a minority of problems have significance for the future.

The accuracy of diagnosis is poor and the information content of the diagnostic labels in common use in primary care is low.

RATIONALE OF CLINICAL PROBLEM SOLVING

There is often more information in the action taken by the physician than in the diagnostic label given for the 95% of biologically less serious illnesses.

Diagnostic information, more often than not, has to be won *de novo* for each new problem.

The primary care team is the central information node in the health care system.

THE ERGONOMICS OF CLINICAL DIAGNOSIS IN AN INTENSIVE CARE WARD

D. E. M. Taylor

Royal College of Surgeons of England, Lincoln's Inn Fields, LONDON WC2A 3PN

Ergonomics is a term of somewhat doubtful etymology formed from analogy with economics. It was originally used in a treatise ascribed to Aristotle entitled " τα οικονομικα " which dealt with household management: on this basis ergonomics may be considered as work management, rather than work efficiency. Therefore this paper will deal with those factors which will assist in optimum patient management from the clinical point of view. The second part of the title also requires explanation and modification, for clinical diagnosis, in the sense of deciding on a unique pathology, is seldom necessary for adequate patient care in an intensive care unit. The number of items of information on which to base a clinical decision in an emergency, or semi-emergency, is limited and there is an almost equally small set of possible therapeutic interventions each of which may be applicable to a number of different causes. Therefore decisions on therapy are taken largely on a judgement of maximal pay-off; that is, a therapeutic intervention is chosen which will be beneficial in a number of given causes of an observed clinical anomaly, and if inappropriate the adverse effects will be minimal. It is not necessary to have a precise clinical diagnosis to reach a decision on patient management. It is with these factors in mind that one must look at the diagnostic process within an ICU. In many ways all types of clinical diagnosis have common features, but it can be studied in its most acute form in an ICU: the most efficient types of information gathering and analysis used in clinical decision making may be more readily assessed in the acute situation of the ICU than in the rather more leisurely general wards or outpatient departments.

SYSTEM ORGANISATION

The traditional concept was that there was a unique relationship between the doctor and the patient; nothing else was considered pertinent to patient management. Although the presence of the nurse was acknowledged, she was considered to be a mere peripheral to the actual decision making processes (Fig. 1a).

The actual work situation consists of a complex net involving not only the patient and the doctor, but also nursing staff and ward equipment and peripheral laboratories: interaction is possible between these items in a large number of combinations (Fig. 1b). The development of the ward system over the centuries has led to unconscious habits of data processing and data presentation which assist heuristic decision making on patient management.

The two basic sources of information for the doctor are the ward chart and the clinical examination. With both of these the major emphasis is placed not on the absolute value of any variable, be it quantitative like blood standard bicarbonate, or qualitative like the degree of pain, but on a comparison with previous estimates and in particular on the detection of consistent time trends (Taylor, 1971). Instantaneous information is of limited utility in decision making except under extreme circumstances such as cardiac arrest; the system has evolved to assist in the recognition of trends, even at the expense of "accuracy" or instantaneous information (Taylor, 1975; Taylor and Whamond, 1975). This involves all human stages in the system, and lack of appreciation of the functions in this process carried out by the nurse has been one factor in the comparatively poor performance of almost totally automated systems of patient care.

UNCONSCIOUS DATA PROCESSING

If a ward chart kept by a nurse is compared to a simultaneous computer-assisted record, more variability appears in the latter than the former (Taylor and Whamond, 1975): indeed computer-assisted records kept over the same period, but with the times of recording separated by 5 minutes, may show little similarity with the chart, although the mean levels and rates of trend are the same on mathematical analysis. This is because of the wide range of normal variation which occurs in the common physiological variables: a co-efficient of variance (SD x 100/mean) of 3-5% occurring with prime variables such as pulse rate and blood pressure (Taylor et al., 1975) and of up to 20% for derived variables such as cardiac output and dP/dt max (Mukhtar and

ERGONOMICS OF CLINICAL DIAGNOSIS

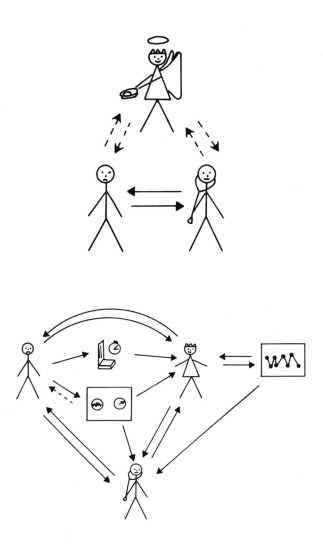

Fig. 1. Interactions in a ward diagnosis situation. (a) Common idea of a simple two way communication between doctor and patient, with only minor interaction with nursing staff. (b) Actual situation with multiple interactions between patient, medical staff, nursing and ancillary staff and equipment. Not shown are outside communications to laboratories and other specialist departments.

Taylor, 1975). These can be observed in both the long and the short term: long term studies of healthy subjects over a 24 hour period have shown that during sleep both pulse rate and arterial pressure have fallen to levels liable to lead to immediate therapeutic intervention if encountered in an intensive care patient (Fig. 2); in the short term of 5 minutes, however, the co-efficient of variance is only about 3% for pulse rate. This distribution, although approximately normal, shows sufficient spread at extreme tails for 5 SDs to be required to encompass 98% of events, giving an effective band-width of 30% of the mean (Taylor et al., 1975).

This accounts for the wide 'noise' element observed on the computer assisted chart, which makes it very difficult to interpret. The chart kept by the nurse is considerably less variable and so, much easier to interpret (Fig. 3): mathematical analysis of the two charts to determine whether changes are influenced by random factors or by trends, have shown that a nurse-kept chart is almost always predominantly affected by trend within 10 entries, whereas the computer-assisted chart is still principally affected by random factors after double the number of entries (Taylor, 1975). A computer-assisted chart showing the same utility for trend detection as the nurses ward chart can be obtained by using a time weighted average, that is, by smoothing (Fig. 4). Investigations have shown that nurses tend to smooth unconsciously, taking into account previous entries with time weighting: if a false chart is substituted when nursing shifts change the new nurse will start entries near to the levels shown and slowly return to the true level over several subsequent entries. Nurses on enquiry freely admit that they frequently take several estimates of a variable, and chart the one nearest to the previous entry. The weighting function unconsciously employed by nurses has an exponential loss of 95% in approximately 8 data points: this means an entry in a $\frac{1}{4}$ hour chart is considering events over the past $1\frac{3}{4}$ hours. When entries are made at longer than hourly intervals the loss of previous information becomes more rapid. This unconscious processing of data assists in clinical decision making, for it delineates trends from the 'noise' of normal biological variations thus providing the type of information on which doctors base management decisions. An experienced consultant or senior registrar is far more likely to order an increase in the rate of blood infusion on the basis of a consistent fall in blood pressure, than on any single absolute value.

Smoothing to accentuate trends is not the only form of unconscious processing; the absolute level of variables may also be biased (Taylor and Whamond, 1975). Where an 'abnormal' level occurs but the overall clinical state is satisfactory, the bias is

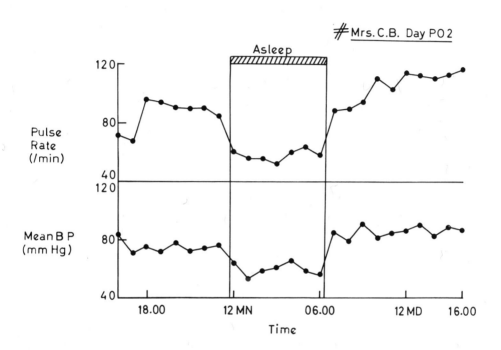

Fig. 2. 24 hr record plotted hourly of pulse rate and mean arterial blood pressure in a patient during the second postoperative day. Despite a satisfactory and stable clinical state throughout, note the wide diurnal fluctuation, particularly the fall in both variables in sleep.

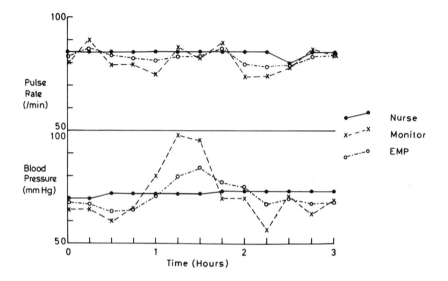

Fig. 3. Quarter hour records kept by a nurse using traditional methods, a computer assisted system with 30 sec time constant, and an exponentially mapped past (decay constant 4 observations) filtering of the computer record. Note the stability of the nurses' observations, compared to the 'true' estimates. Digital filtering gives a closer approximation to the nursing observations.

ERGONOMICS OF CLINICAL DIAGNOSIS

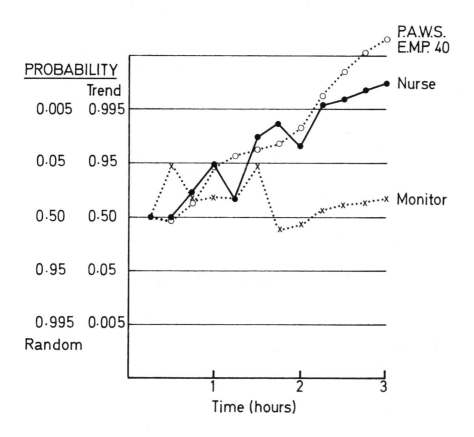

Fig. 4. Probability of differences in a patient chart being due to underlying trends or to random fluctuation (η test). Note that using both the nurses-kept chart and a computer assisted method with a 40 min EMP mean the principal factor causing a difference was trend, whereas using a more normal computer assisted method variation was as much influenced by random fluctuation as trends ever after 3 hours.

towards the 'normal': transient fast arrhythmias are ignored, or
a patient well vaso-dilated but with an adequate circulation has
the blood pressure raised. The latter can amount to about
15 mm Hg, and may account for the fact that although sleeping
blood pressures have been recorded almost since the invention of
the sphygmomanometer, very low pressures of down to 60/40 mm Hg
were only reported in normal subjects after the advent of
automatic recording methods. The converse of a bias away from
normal has also been reported for blood pressure in a patient with
a normotensive oligaemia. Apparent single variables on a ward
chart are probably a compound of multiple variables related to the
same system as that declared; a nurse taking the blood pressure
will unconsciously note skin temperature, skin colour, venous
filling and the presence or absence of sweating (Wolff, 1975),
all of which may modify the value recorded. These biasing
functions also increase the utility of the ward chart, by
increasing the amount of implicit information presented: the
pulse rate and blood pressure provide an overall assessment of
cardiovascular function far beyond what would be possible by an
accurate record of just two variables.

DECISION MAKING

The use made of trend and other clinical data is not so much
directed towards the precise diagnosis which is pathologically
unique, but rather to determining a line of treatment (Dudley,
1968): many 'diagnoses' made are in terms of a recognised symptom
complex rather than a statement of pathological aetiology. For
instance, it is sufficient information to initiate appropriate
treatment merely to know that the patient has suffered a cardiac
arrest; the routine of treatment laid down in most wards is
adequate to cope with such diverse causal aetiologies as
myocardial infarction, oligaemic shock, respiratory inadequacy
with hypoxaemia and renal insufficiency with metabolic acidosis.
Many similar examples were apparent in our intensive care ward,
and to test the applicability of the thesis that in the emergency
situation 'diagnosis' is directed towards establishing a line of
treatment rather than in defining the pathology, all the surgical
deaths in our division of surgery, other than those due to the
progress of proven malignancy where autopsy was obtained, were
analysed over a year, and it was found that, whereas the
pathological diagnosis was correct in under half of the patients,
the treatment was appropriate despite the incorrect clinical
diagnosis in over 80% of patients (Fig. 5). This tends to
confirm that a 'pay-off' philosophy is adopted in clinical
decision meeting, for even where the treatment was inappropriate,
almost without exception its effect on the patient was neutral
rather than deleterious.

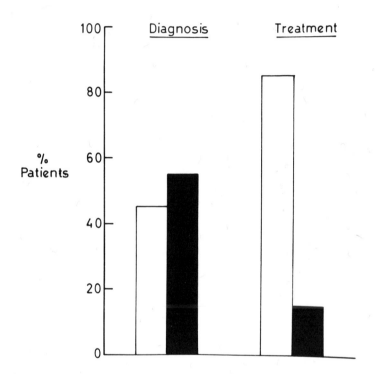

Fig. 5. The "correctness" of diagnosis and treatment
(☐ "correct": ■ "incorrect") in a one-year study of patients in
a large surgical division who died after admission as acute
emergencies. Although the diagnosis on which treatment was
decided was more often wrong than right, in 5 out of 6 patients
the treatment instituted was entirely appropriate to the actual
pathology and only rarely was the treatment completely
inappropriate.

The types of symptom complexes which are looked for tend to reflect disorders of vital body functions, such as circulation, respiration and central nervous activity, and two types of assessment, quantitative and qualitative, are used: each is represented by a different method of data acquisition and of data presentation on the ward chart. The pay-off sought is short term rather than long term and is directed towards the return of the function or variable measured to a 'normal' value.

Quantitative Assessment

Certain physiological variables may be measured accurately by a peripheral laboratory, and thus free of any interaction between the person carrying out the estimation, the patient or the doctor: these include serum electrolytes, acid-base balance and blood gases. Even with these the skilled clinician will balance whether the condition of the patient is consistent with the value recorded on the chart. With many of these variables the normal range for efficient body function is relatively small and therapy is directed towards maintaining clinical chemistry estimates within a normal range; it is an occasional boast of intensive care clinicians that their patients die with their electrolytes normal! All of these variables are usually entered on the chart as a digital value in tabulated form and with 3 significant figures, despite the fact that even with automated methods the accuracy may be only of the order of $\pm$ 5-10%. Therapy is empiric and direct: the method used to correct an anomaly may have little bearing on original cause of the abnormal reading; indeed a potentially lethal biochemical abnormality may be alleviated by inducing a new, but more benign abnormality. For example, a rapid rise in serum potassium, a potentially lethal complication, may occur as a result of intravascular haemolysis or the return of circulation to devitalised muscle; rapid elimination of the excess extracellular potassium from the body is not possible, but it can be translocated into cells by inducing an alkalosis, either respiratory by hyperventilation, or metabolic by the infusion of sodium bicarbonate. The 'pay-off' effect is obvious, a high risk abnormality is replaced by a low risk one, without the necessity of immediately determining the exact aetiology.

Qualitative Assessment

The second class of chart entries are concerned with body functions which can only be assessed in a vague qualitative manner: for example, circulatory sufficiency cannot be precisely defined in terms of blood volume and cardiac output, and even less by blood pressure, pulse rate and central venous pressure. It is

with those estimates that the traditional chart entries of TPR and
BP are concerned and where unconscious pre-processing of data by
staff becomes important. In contrast to the precise numeric
representation of biochemical data, nurse chart entries are
usually graphical in presentation and with scaling which will not
permit representation to better than $\pm$ 5% for pulse rate and BP
and $\pm$ 25% for respiration and CVP. The clinical concern is not
to restore a physiological variable to within narrow and well
defined limits, but rather with the establishment of satisfactorily
clinical function: this is well subserved by the pre-processing
of data which occurs and by the implicit information which is
contained in a data entry point; thus a blood pressure entry of
120/80 mm Hg is principally declaring that the circulation appears
adequate, rather than being an accurate quantitative statement.

Therapy is again decided on a pay-off basis: an inadequate
circulation will be indicated by a low blood pressure entry on the
chart; if this is the principal abnormality treatment is likely to
be by blood transfusion; the latter is the 'correct' therapy if
there is a reduced circulating blood volume from haemorrhage, but
will be equally effective where there is an expanded micro-
circulation, such as in septic shock, where an abnormal blood
volume is produced, or in cardiac power failure, where the
increased diastolic filling pressure will work through the
Starling Law mechanism. In neither of the latter will the
treatment itself correct the basic physiological disturbance, but
provided body function is returned to an optimal state, it
frequently happens that the intrinsic control mechanisms will
overcome the true causal abnormality: exact pathological
diagnosis is often of only academic interest to good patient
management.

CONCLUSIONS

The methods which have evolved of chart keeping and of
interaction between patients and different members of staff are
entirely appropriate to the type of decision making process which
is required within an intensive care situation. The unconscious
data processing and the method of data presentation on the ward
chart work synergistically to improve patient care, by increasing
the probability of early recognition of abnormality and by
directing therapy to restoring optimal function. Ergonomically
we have a very efficient system although from a precise physical
approach it is one which appears highly inaccurate and subjective.
However, the data is presented so that a single datum condenses a
set of information and it is pre-processed so as to minimise
biological 'noise' and accentuate underlying trends: diagnosis is
made from a relatively small set of symptom complexes, rather than

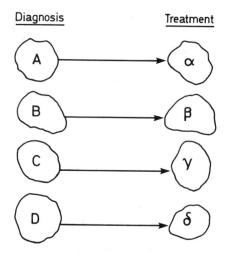

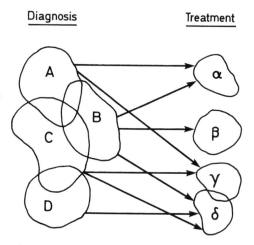

Fig. 6. Venn diagrams to illustrate relationship between "diagnosis" and "treatment". (a) The concept that there are discrete sets of diagnoses each with a specific and unique set of treatment is incorrect; (b) diagnosis sets show considerable overlap and for any single diagnosis set there may be several treatment sets, each of which is equally applicable.

the much larger set of pathological causes; similarly treatment is decided from a set, each member of which is appropriate to more than one diagnosis and with a minimum chance of any inappropriate decision on management having a deleterious effect on prognosis (Fig. 6).

This approach may appear pragmatic and heuristic, but in terms of clinical practice it is firmly based on experience and is effective.

REFERENCES

Dudley, H.A.F. (1968). Lancet, 2, 723.

Mukhtar, A.I. & Taylor, D.E.M. (1975). To be published.

Taylor, D.E.M. (1971). J. Biomed. Eng., Dec., 560.

Taylor, D.E.M. (1975). In "Intensive Care". Ed. Walker, W.F. & Taylor, D.E.M. Published Churchill Livingstone, Edinburgh, London & New York. P. 219.

Taylor, D.E.M., Whamond, Joan S., Hitchings, D.J., Hulliger, M. & Begg, D. (1975). Cardiovasc. Res. In press.

Taylor, D.E.M. & Whamond, Joan S. (1975). European J. Intensive Care. In press.

Wolff, H.S. (1975). In "Intensive Care". Ed. Walker, W.F. & Taylor, D.E.M. Published Churchill Livingstone, Edinburgh. London & New York. P. 31.

INDEX

Abdomen, EMI scanner for, 125
Abortion, 208
Accident and Emergency services, staffing of, 91
Admissions, 209
  computer systems, 220
Alanine transferase, 11, 12
Albumin estimation, 11, 15, 23
Alpha fetoprotein, 48
Amniocentesis, 39
Anencephaly, 48
Anger gamma camera, 73, 75
Angiography of head, 131
Antibiotics in respiratory infections, 257, 259
Aortic blood velocity, 111
Arginosuccinic acid synthetase, 37
Aspartate transferase, 11
Asthma, 172
Australia antigen, 32
Autoanalysers, 31
Automation in pathology, 3-7, 22, 31, 169

Barium meals, 88, 89, 91
Bayes theorem, 212
Bile ducts, dilation of, 88
Biliary tract disease, radiology of, 86
Bilirubin estimation, 15, 23
Biochemical profiles, 9
  accuracy, 18
  current tests, 10
  follow-up of, 16

Biochemical profiling, 9
Blood flow
  rate of, 76
  ultrasonic study of, 69
Blood group serology, 5
Blood transfusion, 5, 32, 185
Blood urea, 32
Body scanning, EMI scanner for, 125
Brain
  abscess, 136
  atrophy, 132
  calcification, 136
  computerised tomography of, 119, 131
  haematoma, 134
  vascular disease of, 134
Brainstem lesions, 159
Brain tumor
  computerised tomography, 122, 132
  detection of, 122
Breast
  radiographic appearance of, 58
Breast cancer,
  detection by mammography, 57
  detection by thermography, 79-84
  screening for, 60

Calcium estimations, 9, 23
Cardiac arrest, 274
Cardiac function
  monitoring of, 176
Cardio-pulmonary by-pass machines, 186

Central venous pressure
   monitoring, 113, 116
Cerebral, See also Brain
Cerebral haemorrhage, 134
Cerebral infarction, 135,
   136, 158
Cerebral oedema, 135, 136
Cerebrovascular disease,
   computerised tomography
   for, 134
Cervical myelopathy, 159, 160
Cervical spondylosis, 149
Chest radiography, as
   screening procedure, 89
Cholecystitis, 86
Cholecystograms, 87
Cholesteatoma, 133
Cholesterol estimation, 9
Chromosomes
  abnormalities, 35, 39
  banding techniques, 42
  obtaining preparations, 41
Cirrhosis of liver, 95
Clinical measurements in
   wards, 165
Clinical problem solving, 251
  information used, 260,
   261, 263
  pathways in, 253
Communication, 172
  importance of, 173
  improvement in, 174
  of results, 193
Computers, 172, 193
  areas of use, 201
  case note storage by, 224
  choice of, 218
  decision making with,
   211-214
  development of systems, 194
  diagnosis by, 211
    comparison with
     clinician, 14
    methods, 212
    results, 213
  direct contact with, 217
  language for, 197
  London Hospital system,
   215-222

Computer (cont'd):
  London Hospital system (cont'd):
    choice of, 218
    cost of, 221
    implementation, 219
    philosophy of, 216
    problems, 222
  -man interaction, 248
  -nurse-patient interaction, 175
  value of, 17
Computer assisted tomography,
   See EMI scanner
Congenital disease, incidence of,
   35
Congenital heart disease, 36
Craniopharyngioma, 133
Creatinine, 11
Cystic fibrosis, 38

Data processing, 5
Day hospitals, 209
Decision making
  by computer, 211-214
  in intensive therapy unit, 274
Demyelinating disease
  diagnosis, 144, 151, 161
Diagnosis
  accuracy of, 36, 254, 256, 275
  computer aided, 211
    comparison with clinicians, 14
    methods, 212
    results, 213
  elements of, 254
  ergonomics contribution to,
   241
  experience of, 243
  in intensive therapy unit,
   267-279
  information used in, 260, 261,
   263, 267
  interactions in, 255, 269
  neurological
    See under Neurological
    diagnosis
  of genetic disorders, 39
  problem solving, 251
  radiation See Radiology
  relationship of components, 255
  relation to therapy, 277, 278

Diagnosis (cont'd):
  training in, 244, 249
  ultrasonic, 63-71
  unconscious data processing, 268
Dialysis, 179
Differential leucocyte counts, 4
Diphtheria, 209
Doctor-patient relationship, 268
Down's syndrome, 38, 42, 48
Drug overdose, 115
Duchenne muscular dystrophy, 45
Dystrophia myotonica, 36

Electroencephalography
  in epilepsy, 108
  in liver disease, 95-106
  in pattern evoked response recording, 139
  normal pattern, 97
  telemetry and video-recording in fits, 107
Electrolytes, estimation, 23, 24, 25, 32
EMI scanner, 90, 170
  accuracy of, 122
  design principles of, 119-130
  for body scanning, 125
  practical experience with, 131-138
Encephalography, 131
Endoscopic retrograde cholangiopancreaticogram, 88
Enzyme defects, 37
Epilepsy, 108
Ergonomics, 241
  definition of, 241, 267
  in medical diagnosis experience of, 243
    in intensive therapy unit, 267

Family file system, 38
Films
  multi-image storage, 231

Finances, 27, 29
  of London Hospital computer system, 221
  of National Health Service, 168
  of pathology, 29, 30
  of radiology, 85, 90
  of radionuclide scanning, 76
  of thermographic screening, 83
Fits
  EEG telemetry and videorecording in, 107
Fluid balance, measurement of, 175
Foetal heart pulsations, 69

Gall stones, 86
Gamma glutamyl transpeptidase, 11, 13
Gas chromatography, 3
Gaucher's disease, 38
Genetic counseling, 35
  value of, 38
Genetic disorders
  antenatal diagnosis, 39
  X-linked, 44
  heterozygote detection, 36
  laboratory diagnosis of, 35-53
Genetic risks, 36
Glucose-6-phosphate dehydrogenase, 37

Haemangioma of orbit, 137
Haemodialysis, 179
Haemodynamic assessment by transcutaneous aortovelography, 109-117
Haemoglobin estimation, 4
Hare lip, 36
Head, computerised tomography of, 119
Health information systems, 207-210
Heart, computerised tomography of, 130
Hepatic coma, 95
Hepatitis, 95
Hereditary spino-cerebellar ataxia, 151
Histidinaemia, 45
Histopathology, 4

Homocystinuria, 45
Hospitals, length of stay in, 208
Huntington's chorea, 36
Hydrocephalus, 132
Hyperparathyroidism, 9
Hypovolaemic shock, transcutaneous aortovelography in, 113
Hypoxanthine guanine phosphoribosyl transferase, 37

Information retrieval, 195
Infra-red radiation emitted by skin, 79
Intensive therapy units, 186
  decision making in, 274
  ergonomics of clinical diagnosis, 267-279
  fluid balance measurement in, 175
  haemodynamic assessment with transcutaneous aortovelography, 109-117
  nurse-patient-computer interaction in, 175
  patient assessment in, 276
  pressure recording in, 176
  psychological needs of patients, 187
  staff training, 177, 189
Intracranial calcification, 136

Jaundice
  obstructive, 87

Kidney, computerised tomography of, 126
Kodak Retnar system, 226

Laboratories
  centralisation, 19-28, 29
  rationalisation of, 27, 28
Lactate dehydrogenase, 12
Lesch-Nyhan syndrome, 37
Liver, computerised tomography of, 126
Liver disease, electroencephalography in, 95-106

Liver failure, 95, 97, 102
  clinical features, 104
Liver necrosis, 95
London Hospital computer system, 215-222
  choice of, 218
  cost of, 221
  implementation, 219
  philosophy of, 216
  problems, 222
Lungs, computerised tomography of, 126, 130
Lysosomal acid phosphatase, 37

Machines, interaction with man, 248
Macrofiches, 227
Mammography, 57-61
  image enhancement in, 59
  in disease screening, 60
  normal appearance, 58
  technique, 58
Man-machine interface, 248
Massachusetts Utility Medical Program Systems (MUMPS), 197
  advantages and disadvantages of, 202
  areas of use, 201
  development of, 204
Measles, 209
Medical linguistics for computers, 197
Meningioma, 149, 150
Metabolic disorders, antenatal diagnosis, 45
Microfilm systems, 223-229
  storage, 226
    computers in, 224, 228
    possibilities of, 228
Multi-image storage, 231-237
Multiple sclerosis
  diagnosis, 139, 146, 147, 148, 159, 160, 162
  optic nerve plaques in, 145
Muscular dystrophy, 38, 45
Myocardial infarction, 274
  computer diagnosis, 14
  mortality rate, 208
  transcutaneous aortovelography in, 113

National Health Service, 168, 172
Neuritis
  optic, 144, 145
  retrobulbar, 146, 161
Neurological diagnosis
  peripherally evoked spinal cord potentials in, 155
  visually evoked cortical potentials in, 139-153
Neurosurgical units, 32
5-Nucleotidase, 11
Nurses and nursing
  basic and technical, 185-189
  in intensive care units, 175, 186, 270
  -patient-computer interaction, 175

Operative cholangiography, 87
Optic atrophy, congenital, 151
Optic nerve plaques, 145
Optic neuritis, 143, 144, 145
Orbital disease, 136
Oxford Record Linkage Study, 173

Pancreas, computerised tomography, 126
Pathology, 169
  automation in, 3-7, 22, 31, 169
  cost-benefit comparisons, 30
  data processing, 5
  financial factors, 27, 29, 30
  laboratory centralisation, 19-28
  new tests, 30
  routine and non-routine tests, 32
  specialised analyses, 29
Patients
  admissions, 209
  assessment in intensive care unit, 276
  interaction with machines, 179
  length of stay in hospital, 208
  -nurse-computer interaction, 175
  psychological needs of, 187
  training in renal dialysis, 181

Pattern revoked response recording
  averaging method, 141
  clinical testing, 141
  in multiple sclerosis, 144, 145, 146, 147, 148
  latency of, 143
  in neurological diagnosis, 139
  in progressive spastic paraplegia, 148, 149
Percutaneous transhepatic cholangiogram, 88
Perinatal mortality, 208
Peripherally evoked spinal cord potentials, 155
  in neurological disease, 157
  method, 155
  normal, 156
Phenylketonuria, 37, 38
Phosphorus estimation, 23
Physics, 26
Potassium estimation, 11
Pregnancy, disease screening during, 39, 53
Problem solving, 251
  information used, 260, 261, 263
  pathways, 253
Progressive spastic paraplegia, 148, 149
Protein bound iodine, 13
Protein estimations, 23

Radiographers, role of, 91
Radiology, 169
  accuracy of, 18
  cost of, 85, 90
  filing systems, 224
  in diagnosis, 57-61
  multi-image storage, 231
  perspectives in, 85-92
Radionuclide imaging, 73-77
  Anger gamma camera, 73, 75
  cost of, 76
  scanners, 73
Radiopharmaceuticals, 74, 76
Records, 261
  computer storage, 224
  content of, 262
  microfilms, 223
  multi-image storage, 231-237

Register for the ascertainment and prevention of inherited disease, 38
Renal dialysis
  at home, 181
  patient-machine interaction, 179
  patient training in, 181
  safety precautions, 183
  support for patient, 182
  units, 32
Renal failure, 106, 179
Respirators, 186
Respiratory infections
  antibiotics in, 257, 259
  diagnosis, 257, 258
Results, co-ordination and communication of, 193
Retrieval systems, 195
  microfilms in, 223
Retrobulbar neuritis, 146, 161
Rheumatoid arthritis, 15

Screening for disease, 9-16, 167
  biliary tract disease, 86
  biochemical profiles, 9, 18
  breast cancer, 83
  chest radiography, 89
  during pregnancy, 39, 53
  essential tests, 11
  mammography in, 60
  problems, 17
  thermography in, 83
Shock, 274
  transcutaneous aortovelography in, 113
Skin temperature, 79
Social workers, 171
Sodium estimation, 11
Spina bifida, 36, 48
Spinal cord potentials, peripherally evoked See Peripherally evoked spinal cord potentials
Spleen, computerised tomography of, 126
Spondylosis, 149, 159
Strokes, 136

Tay Sachs disease, 38, 45
Technetium, 74
Therapy
  laboratory tests and, 31
  relationship with diagnosis, 277, 278
Thermography for breast cancer, 79-84,
  criteria, 80
  evaluation, 80, 81
  screening, 83
Thyroid gland, 13
Tomography, computerised See under EMI scanner
Tomography, transverse axial See EMI scanner
Transcutaneous aortovelography
  clinical experience with, 112
  comparison with other measurements, 112
  haemodynamic assessment by, 109-117
  interpretation of, 111
  method, 110
  principles of, 109
Transverse axial tomography See EMI scanner
Triglyceride assay, 9
Tunnel vision, 90

Ultrasonic diagnostics, 63-71
  brightness, 67
  Doppler systems, 68
  gray-scale scanning, 68, 90
  of blood flow, 69
  of foetal heart pulsations, 69
  pulse-echo systems, 63
  resolution, 65
  sound spectrograph in, 69
Urea estimation, 11, 23

Valearic acid
  EEG and, 104
Videorecording of EEG, 107
Viral hepatatis, 95

Xero radiography, 59